Spina Bifida and Craniosynostosis - New Perspectives and Clinical Applications

Edited by Branislav Kolarovszki, Raffaella Messina and Valeria Blè

Published in London, United Kingdom

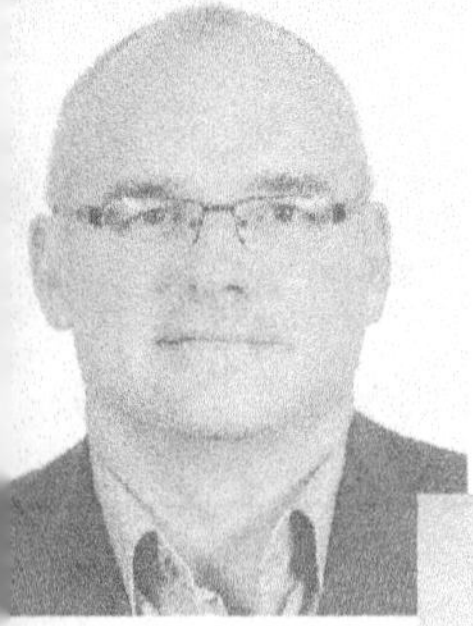
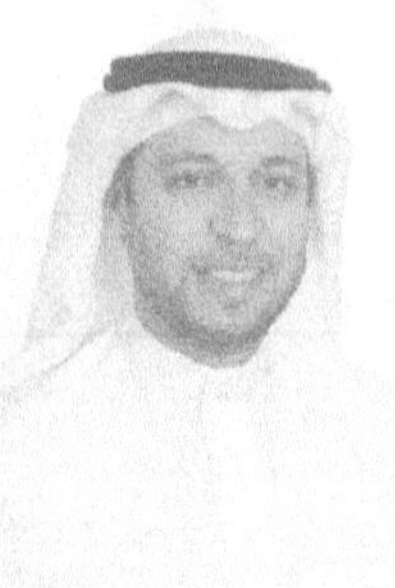
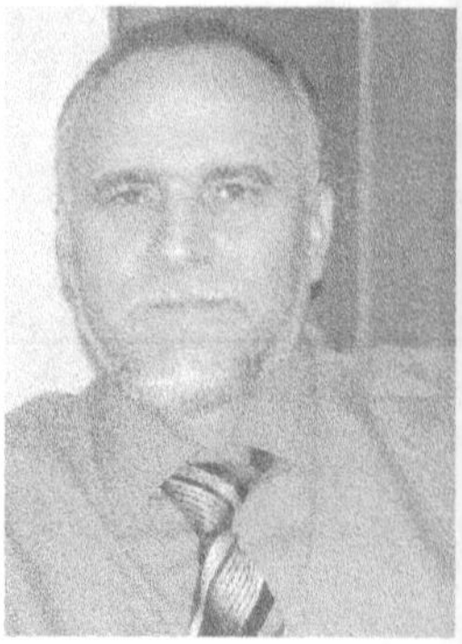
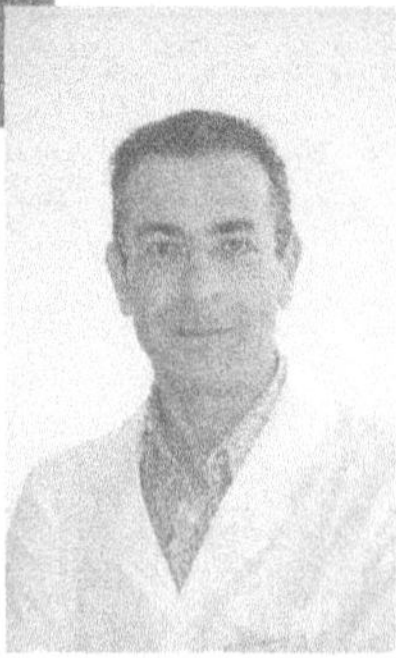
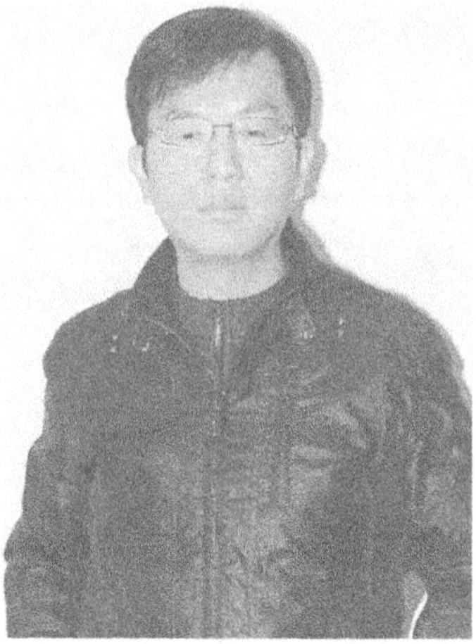
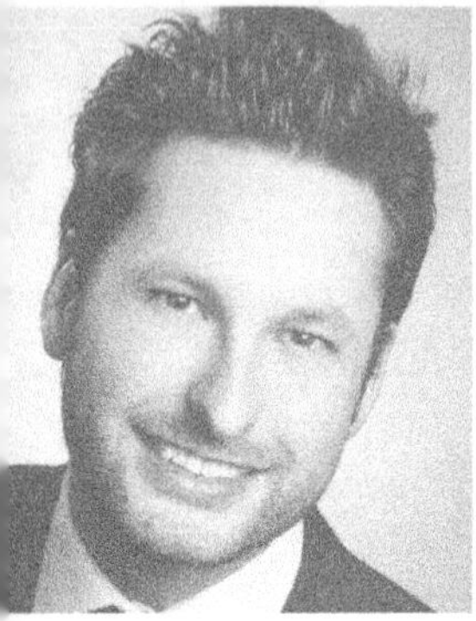
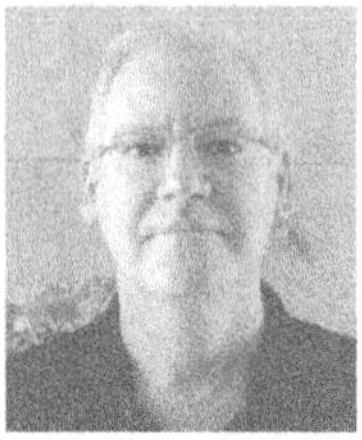

IntechOpen

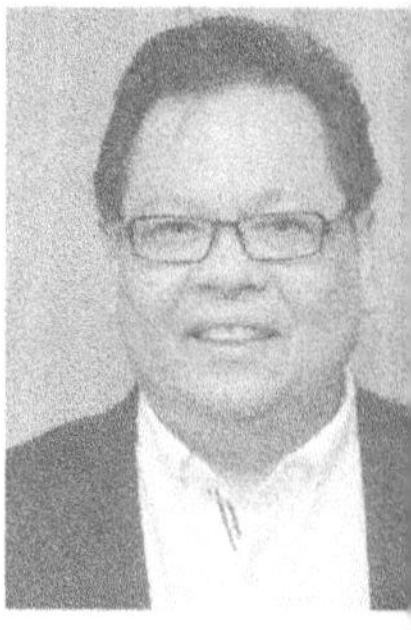
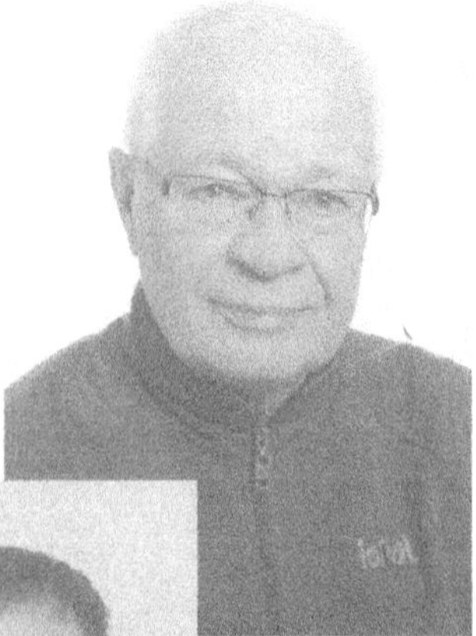
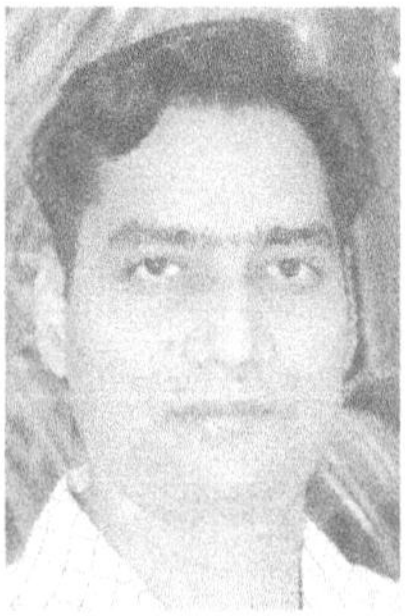
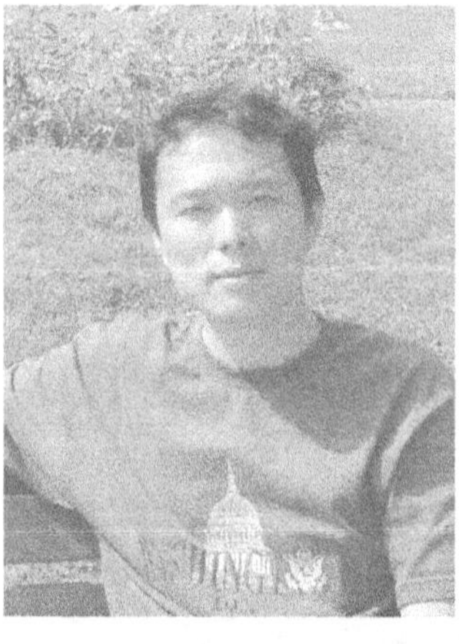
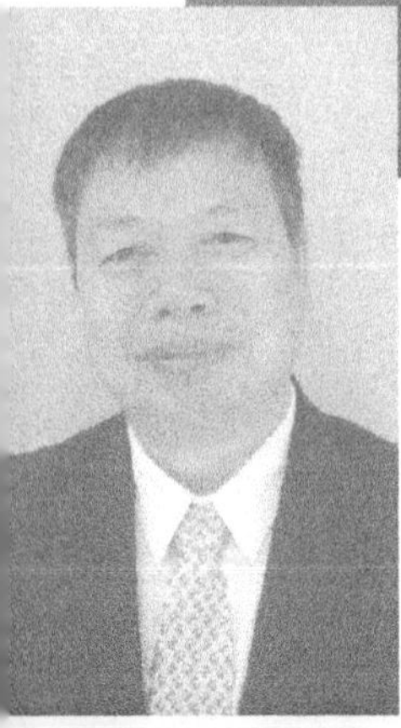
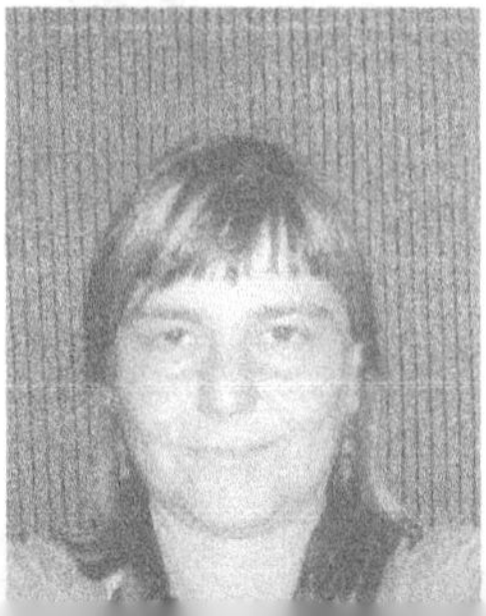

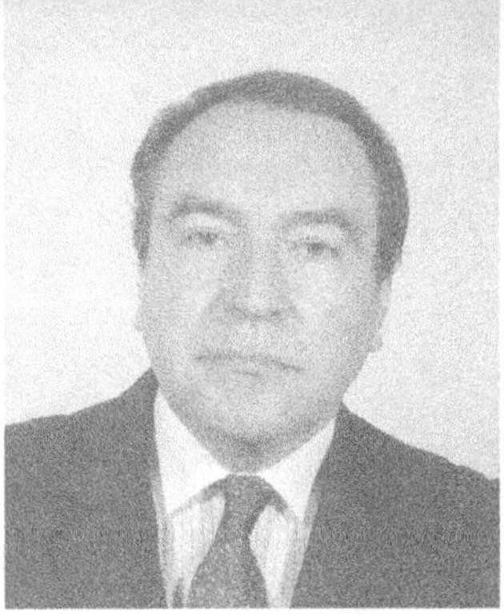
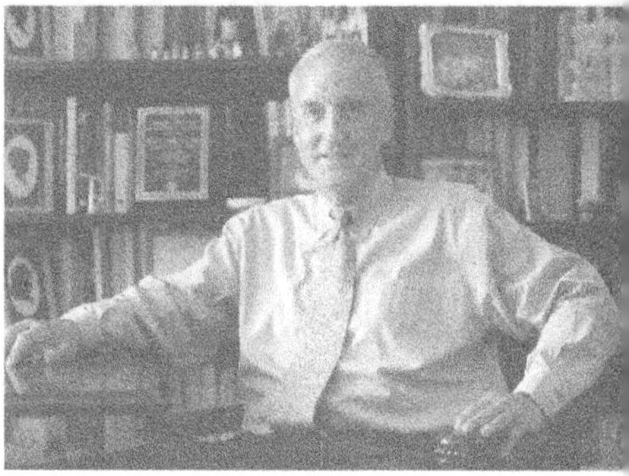
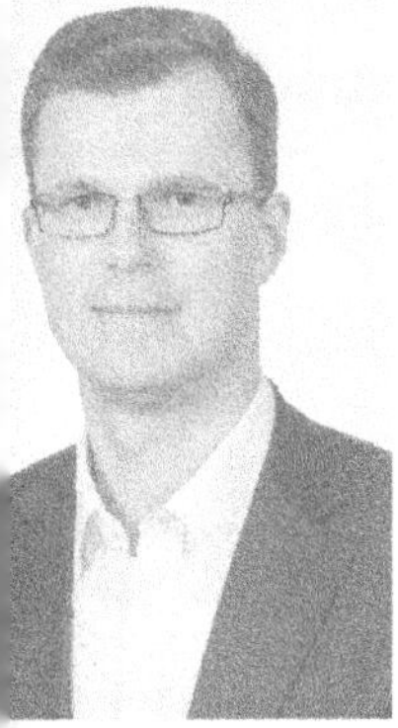
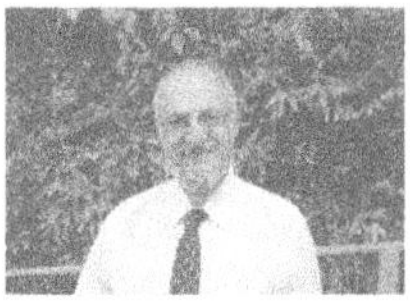
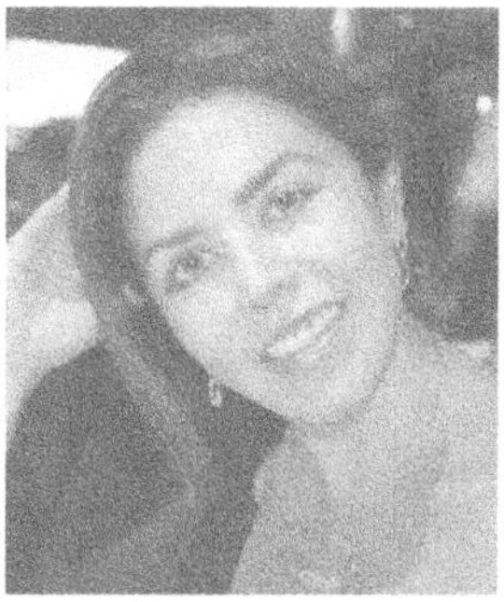

Supporting open minds since 2005

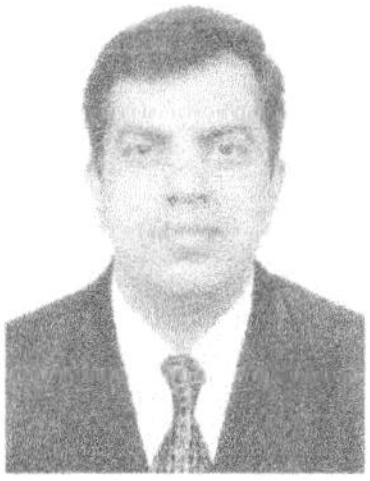
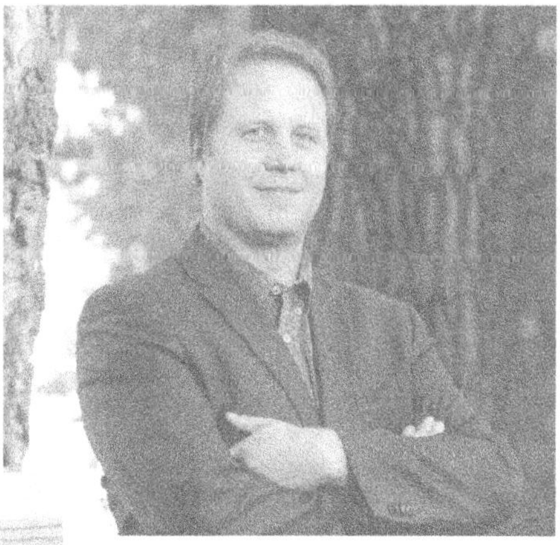
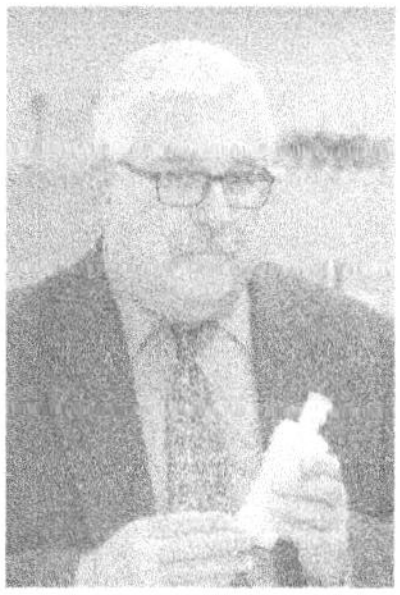
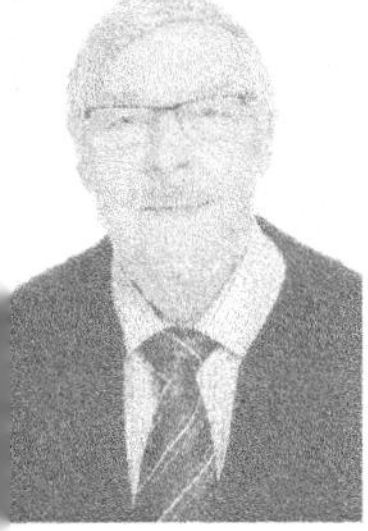
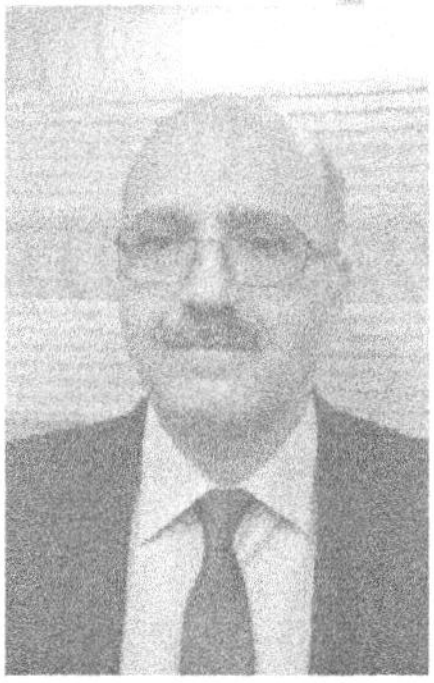
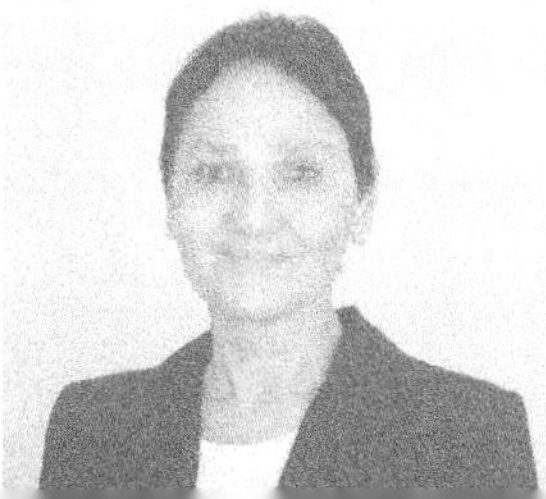
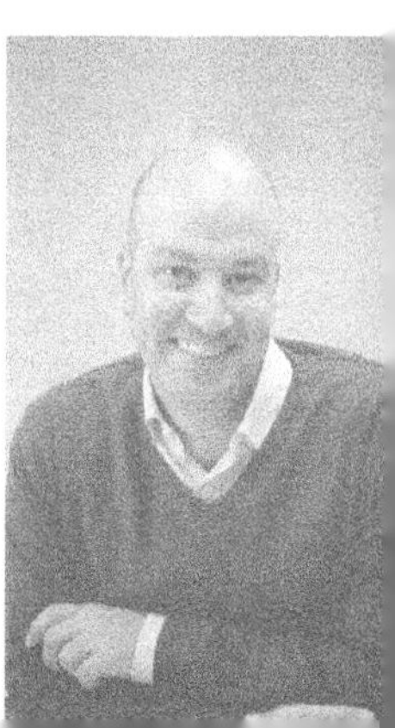

Spina Bifida and Craniosynostosis - New Perspectives and Clinical Applications
http://dx.doi.org/10.5772/intechopen.77598
Edited by Branislav Kolarovszki, Raffaella Messina and Valeria Blè

Contributors
David García-Mato, Javier Pascau, Santiago Ochandiano, Khairul Bariah Chi Adam, Firdaus Hariri, Lee Chee Wei, Nazer Berahim, Kathiravan Perumal, Mohd Faizal Abdullah, Adrián Gutiérrez-González, José Iván Robles-Torres, Daniel García-Sánchez, Ana C. Belzarena, Roselle Okubo, Claudio Silveri, Diego José Caycedo, Marcela Cabal Castro, René Opšenák, Branislav Kolarovszki, Romana Richterová, Juraj Sutovsky, Luis Fernando Santacruz

First published in London, United Kingdom, 2021 by IntechOpen
IntechOpen is the global imprint of INTECHOPEN LIMITED, registered in England and Wales, registration number: 11086078, 5 Princes Gate Court, London, SW7 2QJ, United Kingdom
Printed in Croatia

British Library Cataloguing-in-Publication Data
A catalogue record for this book is available from the British Library

Additional hard and PDF copies can be obtained from orders@intechopen.com

Spina Bifida and Craniosynostosis - New Perspectives and Clinical Applications
Edited by Branislav Kolarovszki, Raffaella Messina and Valeria Blè
p. cm.
Print ISBN 978-1-83962-950-1
Online ISBN 978-1-83962-951-8
eBook (PDF) ISBN 978-1-83962-952-5

Meet the editors

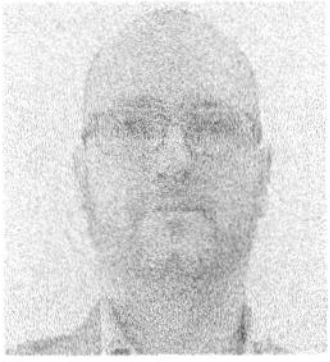

Assoc. Prof. Branislav Kolarovszki, MD, Ph.D., is the head of the Clinic of Neurosurgery, Jessenius Faculty of Medicine in Martin, Comenius University in Bratislava, University Hospital in Martin, Slovakia. For many years he deals with the issues of pediatric neurosurgery, especially hydrocephalus, spina bifida, and craniosynostosis. He published the results of his work in many scientific journals and monographs. He actively participates in congresses, including invited lectures on pediatric neurosurgery. Dr. Kolarovszki is a member of editorial boards and a reviewer of many medical journals. He is currently the first vice-dean of the Jessenius Faculty of Medicine.

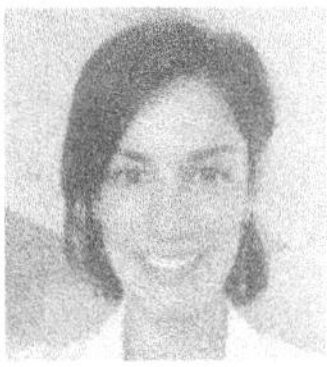

Dr. Raffaella Messina is an Italian board-certified neurosurgeon. She was trained in neurosurgery at the University Hospital of Bari, Italy. She has held a fellowship in pediatric neurosurgery at the IRCCS Institute for Treatment and Research - Bambino Gesù Children's Hospital, Rome. She is currently pursuing a Ph.D. in Neurosciences and has been an assistant professor at the University of Bari "Aldo Moro," Italy, since 2010. Her major field of interest is pediatric neurosurgery, in which she has focused her main scientific activity. She had the opportunity to improve her surgical skills and to achieve board certification for the European Society for Pediatric Neurosurgery (ESPN), attending the three-year cycle of ESPN.

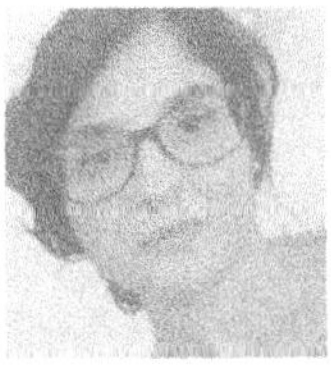

Dr. Valeria Blé is an Italian board-certified neurosurgeon. She was trained in neurosurgery at the University Hospital of Bari, Italy, and was an observer in pediatric neurosurgery at Hôpital Femme Mère Enfant, Lyon, France, and fellow at the IRCCS Institute for Treatment and Research - Bambino Gesu Children's Hospital, Rome. She is a consultant neurosurgeon in the University Hospital in Bari, Italy. Her major field of interest is pediatric neurosurgery, and she is currently taking a post-graduate course in Pediatric Neurosurgery.

Contents

Preface XI

Section 1
Spina Bifida 1

Chapter 1 3
Etiology and Pathophysiology of the Spina Bifida
by René Opšenák, Romana Richterová and Branislav Kolarovszki

Chapter 2 27
Management of Pediatric Patients with Spina Bifida
by Romana Richterová, Branislav Kolarovszki and René Opšenák

Chapter 3 57
Surgical Treatment of Neural Tube Defects
by Juraj Šutovský

Chapter 4 77
Urologic Implications and Management in Spina Bifida
by Adrián Gutiérrez-González, José Iván Robles-Torres and Daniel García-Sánchez

Chapter 5 91
Orthopedic Approach to Spina Bifida
by Roselle C. Okubo, Claudio Silveri and Ana C. Belzarena

Section 2
Craniosynostosis 107

Chapter 6 109
New Technologies to Improve Surgical Outcome during Open-Cranial Vault Remodeling
by David García-Mato, Javier Pascau and Santiago Ochandiano

Chapter 7 129
Craniofacial Corrective Surgery in Syndromic Craniosynostosis
by Khairul Bariah Chi Adam, Firdaus Hariri, Wei Lee Chee, Kathiravan Purmal, Mohd Faizal Abdullah and Nazer Berahim

Chapter 8 147
Telescoping with Multiple Revolution Cranial Osteotomies in Patients with Simple Craniosynostosis
by Diego José Caycedo, Marcela Cabal Castro and Luís Fernando Santacruz

Preface

This book about pediatric neurosurgery deals with spina bifida and craniosynostosis. It offers the reader an overview of the diseases with emphasis on the application of new methods and treatment strategies in daily clinical practice.

Spina bifida is a neurodevelopmental disorder and one of the most common congenital malformations. Although patient survival rates have improved over the last decades, neural tube defects are still a substantial cause of morbidity in children. Survival and quality of life are associated with access to proper medical and surgical treatment as well as community support systems. This multidisciplinary approach is the reason for improved patient outcomes in quality of life and life expectancy in the last 50 years. Due to the many complications of this complex health issue, there is an essential need for a multidisciplinary approach to monitor, prevent, and treat possible complications that negatively impact functionality, life quality, and survival. Parents and close caregivers have a crucial role in the entire multidisciplinary team. Raising the child in a caring environment could help them develop into young adults able to go to school and work, find and use transportation, live on their own, and have healthy relationships.

Craniosynostosis is caused by the premature closure of one or more skull sutures. It causes a deformity of the baby's head, which is often visible after birth or in early infancy. The impulse for the growth of a child's head is the growth of the brain. In the case of craniosynostosis, the growth of the skull is limited and deformed, which can negatively affect the growth and development of the brain. Due to this, craniosynostosis cannot be considered only as a cosmetic matter, especially in severe forms or in the case of premature closure of several skull sutures. The diagnosis of craniosynostosis is based on the clinical picture, anthropometric examination with craniometric scan, X-ray, CT, and MRI examination of the skull and brain. The treatment for craniosynostosis is surgical, the aim of which is to modify the shape of the skull. In the case of severe forms, especially syndromological craniosynostosis, the aim is to prevent secondary brain damage. In the past, only open remodeling techniques had been used in the surgical treatment of craniosynostosis. Currently, endoscopic methods with subsequent remodeling treatment with a cranial orthosis are increasingly used.

I believe that this book will be useful for experts from several medical disciplines, especially pediatricians, neonatologists, neurologists, neurosurgeons, maxillofacial surgeons, orthopedists, and urologists.

Branislav Kolarovszki, M.D., Ph.D.
Associate Professor,
Clinic of Neurosurgery,
Jessenius Faculty of Medicine in Martin,
Comenius University in Bratislava,
University Hospital Martin,
Slovakia

Dr. Raffaella Messina and Dr. Valeria Blé
University of Bari Medical School "Aldo Moro",
Bari, Italy

Section 1

Spina Bifida

Chapter 1

Etiology and Pathophysiology of the Spina Bifida

René Opšenák, Romana Richterová and Branislav Kolarovszki

Abstract

The spina bifida is a congenital anomaly that results in an abnormal formation of the spine and the spinal cord. The two dominant types of spinal dysraphism are based on appearance - open spina bifida if the lesion is visible and closed spina bifida if the lesion is not visible on the body surface. These conditions lead to a different spectrum of neurological effects according to the degree of neurulation disruption. The prevalence of neural tube defects has different rates among different ethnicity, geography, gender, and countries. Genetic, nutritional and environmental factors play a role in the etiology and pathogenesis of the spina bifida. Congenital anomalies in the vast majority concern children living in the early neonatal period who have important medical, social or educational needs. The lifetime cost of a child born with the spina bifida is estimated at over €500,000.

Keywords: neural tube defects, spina bifida, spinal dysraphism, etiology, pathophysiology, meningomyelocele

1. Introduction

Spinal dysraphism encompasses congenital problems that result in an abnormal bony formation of the spine and the spinal cord. This congenital pathology is caused by the maldevelopment of the ectodermal, mesodermal, and neuroectodermal tissues. The spina bifida is a congenital anomaly that arises from incomplete development of the neural tube. It is commonly used as a nonspecific term referring to any degree of neural tube closure. The two dominant types of spinal dysraphism are based on the appearance – spina bifida aperta if the lesion is visible and spina bifida occulta if the lesion is not visible [1]. Common manifestations are meningocele, myelomeningocele, lipomeningocele, lipomyelomenigocele, myeloschisis, and rachischisis [1]. Spinal neural tube defects basicaly exist in two forms – open and closed spinal dysraphism. The most simple form with minimal involvement of nervous tissue is closed dysraphism (spina bifida occulta) where the vertebral defect is hidden. More severe open spinal dysraphisms (spina bifida aperta) mostly represented by meningocele or myelomeningocele result in various degrees of neurological deficit according to affected spine level, extent of lesion and amount of structures involved (**Figure 1**). In this defect there is a communication between nerve tissue and external environment leading to exposure to amniotic fluid and later leads to high risk of infection. Defect can be covered by a thin membrane. The exposed neural tissue degenerates *in utero,* resulting in

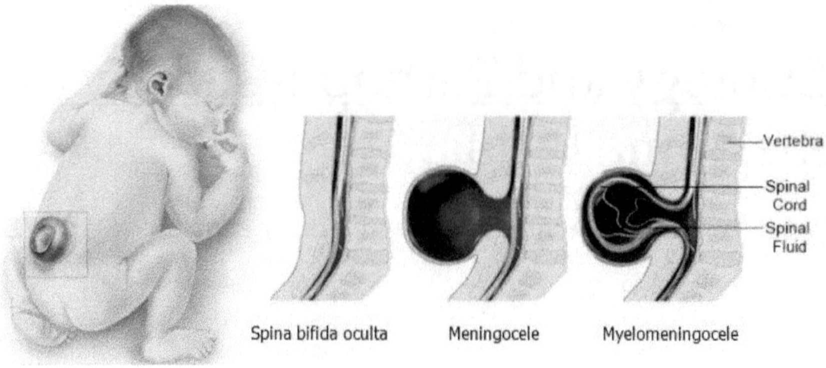

Figure 1.
Types of spinal dysraphism (public domain, source: wikipedia.org).

neurological deficit that varies with level of the lesion. The vertebrae at the level of the lesion lacks neural arches, and so are incomplete dorsally. Spina bifida is commonly associated with several other developmental abnormalities which makes a multidisciplinary medical plan paramount to survival and positive outcomes. The spina bifida correlates with cutaneous conditions such as port-wine stain, hemangioma, hypertrichosis, fibroma pendulum, pigmentary nevus, lipoma, dermal sinus, and deviation of the gluteal furrow [2]. Motor and sensory neurological deficit is inconsistent. The result of nerve structures involvement is usually paraparesis – weakness of lower extremities which in more severe degrees leads to impaired walking or immobility. In patients with severe forms of spina bifida degree of disability strongly correlates with axial level of the lesion [3]. Long term 40-years follow-up of 117 children in the United Kingdom who underwent surgical repair during the 1960s and 1970s showed only 17% of survivors with high level of lesion (above T11) and these patients have higher risk of pressure sores and significantly lower possibility to become community walker. Survival in patients with lesion below L3 vertebra was 61%. Loss of skin sensitivity increases the risk of development of pressure sores what makes frequent skin control necessary. Incontinence of stools and urine is very frequent as well as orthopedic complications, such as contractures, talipes, dislocation of the hip joint, kyphosis and scoliosis. Patients with open forms of spina bifida often display also Chiari II malformation (herniation of the hindbrain) and hydrocephalus that could also require shunting procedure. The mobility and the need for care can be predicted from the neurological deficit. [4]. The lifetime cost of a child born with the spina bifida is estimated at over €500,000, of which 37% comprises direct medical costs with the remaining being indirect costs including special educational and caregiver needs, and loss of employment potential. The direct medical cost for spina bifida patients throughout their life is very high. The most significant amount of financial cost consumpts initial diagnosis and early treatment, inpatient care and the treatment of comorbidities in adult life. The indirect lifetime cost in these patients is even higher due to great impact of their increased overall morbidity. The results from the economic evaluations demonstrate that folic acid fortification in food and pre-conception folic acid consumption are cost-effective ways to reduce the incidence of neural tube defects [5, 6]. Considering all possible medical and economic consequences of the issue of diagnosis of spina bifida, there is an emerging need for clarification of exact etiology and pathophysiological mechanisms with emphasis on possible primary prevention, as well as early and effective treatment of spina bifida and also all upcoming complications.

2. Epidemiology

The prevalence of neural tube defects has different rates among different ethnicity, geography, gender, and also countries. The prevalence is higher among Whites as compared to Blacks and females as compared to males [7]. Asia has more rate of neural tube defects than western countries due to low socio-economic status of eastern countries directly affecting the economic burden and negligence over the folic acid as a part of multivitamin supplementation [8]. Worldwide data show place to place-variation of the prevalence rate assumed to be due to low standard health care facilities though the exact mechanism is still unknown. The eastern Mediterranean region exhibited high variability with a swat, Pakistan having 124 cases per 10000 births. The prevalence in the African region ranges from 5.2 to 75.4 per 10000 births, the European region ranges from 1.3 to 35.9 per 10000, and American region ranges from 1.4 to 27.9 cases per 10000. Most WHO member states (120/194) did not have any data on the prevalence of neural tube defects. As the prevalence estimates vary widely, efforts need to be stepped up to monitor neural tube disorders, especially in developing countries. The folic acid supplementation and increasing the quality of the population's diet are important factors in the prevention [9]. A study from Los Angeles showed that the rate of anencephaly and exencephaly is more than spina bifida. But normally, it is supposed that the spina bifida is more common than anencephaly. Same-sex twins had a higher incidence of neural tube defects as well as higher mortality. The study verifies the same etiology between neural tube defects and monozygotic twins. The main role here is played by the common susceptibility to environmental factors [7]. The rate of neural tube defects is more common in twins than singleton and in monozygotic twins than dizygotic twins. The spina bifida most frequently affects lumbosacral spinal level. Only about 0–5% of cases occur in the cervical spine, 5–10% in the thoracic spine, 20–30% in the thoracolumbar junction, 20–30% in the lumbar, 30–50% in the lumbosacral level and 5–15% in the sacral spine [10]. Altogether cervicothoracic spinal dysraphisms are rare, with an incidence of only 1–6,5% [11]. Myelomeningocele occurs in approximately 1 in 1200 to 1400 births. 60% of those children are community ambulators, and 80% are socially continent. The incidence is not higher in any specific ethnic group, but females have a slightly higher incidence in comparison with males [12]. An increased risk of recurrence has been reported of about 3–8% after one affected pregnancy or maternal history of the defect and the risk worsens with an increasing number of affected children [13]. Researchers performed a study in northern China that showed that the recurrence risk in neural tube defects in subsequent pregnancies was 1.7%, which was higher than in the United States. The recurrence rate of neural tube defects was approximately 5-times higher than the overall prevalence in the same region of northern China [14]. The risk of recurrence in myelomeningocele was reported 2–5% in the United States. These data suggest that the genetic basis of closed defects may be same as the basis for myelomeningocele in some families [15]. Another study showed that the recurrence rate has been approximately 2–3% in consecutive pregnancies. Higher incidence rates were reported in females, increased maternal age, and lower socio-economic status. Latin Americans were the most affected population in the United States. Females are affected up to 3- to 7-times more than males [16]. The observed prevalence of the spina bifida varies globally and is largely influenced by differences in surveillance methods, prenatal diagnosis and elective termination policies, and folic acid fortification of staple foods in a given country or region. The spina bifida is more common in countries where there is no legislation providing for the mandatory enrichment of the diet with folic acid in order to reduce its prevalence. African data were scarce, but needed, as many African nations are beginning to adopt folic acid legislation [9, 17, 18]. Ultrasound screening has a major impact on the epidemiology of the spina bifida. The prenatal detection rate of spina bifida is high, and most cases of spina bifida are isolated and have a normal karyotype [19]. Omission of elective terminations clearly underestimates prevalence and may bias risk estimations in etiologic studies. Compared with women who delivered liveborn/stillborn infants with neural tube defects, women who electively terminated neural tube defects-affected pregnancies were disproportionately white, were more highly educated, had higher incomes, and used vitamins containing folic acid more often [20]. The European network of population-based registries for epidemiological surveillance of congenital anomalies (EUROCAT), collects data on pregnancy terminations in addition to live and stillbirths, generating particularly comprehensive prevalence data for neural tube defects and other malformations. During four years (2003 to 2007), this register reports an overall prevalence of serious congenital anomalies of 23.9 per 1,000 live births. As many as 80% of children with severe congenital anomalies were born alive. The mortality of these children in the first week of life was 2.5%. The abortion was performed after prenatal diagnosis in 17.6% of cases. Congenital anomalies mainly concern newborns with specific medical and social care needs. The prevalence of chromosomal abnormalities was 3.6 per 1,000 live births. Their presence led to a 28% incidence of stillbirths or their diagnosis conditioned 48% of all terminations. The most common non-chromosomal subgroups were congenital heart defects, limb anomalies, nervous system disorders and urinary system anomalies. In 2004, perinatal mortality associated with congenital anomaly was 0.93 per 1000 births, and terminations of pregnancy following prenatal diagnosis 4.4 per 1000 births, with considerable country variation. Primary prevention of congenital anomalies in the population based on controlling environmental risk factors is a crucial policy priority, including pre-conceptional care and whole population approaches [21].

3. Etiology

The development of nervous system is an embryonal process called neurulation. The primary neurulation is the first phase and includes the closure of the neural tube and thus forming brain and spinal cord. The second phase comprises formation of sacral and coccygeal segment and occurs around 26th day of gestation. Spina bifida is an incomplete closure of dorsal spinal structures and usually happens to appear between 17th to 30th postconceptional day [3]. The etiology of spinal dysraphism is multifactorial [22]. Although no clear etiology is known to result in either the open or closed forms, some regional adverse factors have been reported, primarily involving the mother at conception and early pregnancy. **Table 1** lists potential risk factors that are usually considered to be neural tube defects. Grewal et al. report in their study that maternal intake of the alcohol increased the risk for d-transposition of the great arteries, neural tube defects, and multiple cleft lip with or without cleft palate in infants. Smoking in this study was associated with a lower risk of neural tube defects [23]. Positive associations are observed between spina bifida and caffeine consumption and each caffeine source except caffeinated tea, which showed a negative association with the spina bifida. The association between caffeine consumption and anencephaly differed by maternal race and ethnicity. No dose effect of caffeine consumption was found [24]. Plasma levels of folate and vitamin B12 are independent risk factors for the occurrence of neural tube defects. This fact suggests that the enzyme methionine synthase is involved in the etiology of neural tube defects. The surprising finding is that folate and vitamin B12 levels, considered sufficient, continued to be a risk factor for an increased incidence of this defects. This finding is an incentive to re-evaluate daily doses of folate as well as

Maternal nutrition	Other maternal factors	Environmental factors
Alcohol and caffeine use	Smoking	Ambient air pollution
Insufficient folate intake	Low socio-economic status	Indoor air pollution
Low dietary quality	Infections and hyperthermia	Nitrate-related compounds
Elevated glycemic load	Pregestational diabetes	Organic solvents
Low methionine and zinc intake	Pregestational obesity	Pesticides
Low serum choline level	Psychosocial stress	Polycyclic hydrocarbons
Low vitamin B12 and C level	Valproic acid use	Disinfectant in drinking water

Table 1.
Potential risk factors for neural tube defects (according to [3]).

vitamin B12 [25]. The higher quality of the diet of expectant mothers is associated with a reduced incidence of neural tube defects. It is dietary approaches that could further reduce the risk of serious birth defects and complement existing efforts to promote the use of multivitamins during pregnancy [26]. Yazdy et al. refer that high insulin intake is risk factor for genesis of neural tube defects [27]. Results from experimental animals have suggested a role for methionine, an essential amino acid, in normal closure of the neural tube. Shaw et al. observed an approximately 30–40% reduction in neural tube defect-affected pregnancies among women whose average daily dietary intake of methionine was above the lowest quartile of intake. These reductions in neural tube defect risk were observed for both anencephaly and spina bifida, remained after adjustment for maternal race, ethnicity and education; and were observed irrespective of maternal level of folate intake [28]. Shaw al. observed elevated risk of neural tube defects associated with lower levels of total choline, and reduced risks with its higher level [29]. In the systematic review, Ray et al. report a moderate association between low maternal B12 status and the risk of fetal neural tube defects [30]. Studies report a reduction in the risk of neural tube disorders in infants and fetuses when mothers taking zinc in the preconception period. However, it has not been established whether the combination of nutrients or zinc alone is associated with a reduced incidence of neural tube disorders [31]. Maternal hyperthermia in early pregnancy is associated with increased risk for neural tube defects and may be a human teratogen [32]. Similarly, lower socio-economic status and residence in a socio-economic status-lower neighborhood increased the risk of neural tube defect-affected pregnancy [33]. Although the excess risk for birth defects among children of mothers with diabetes mellitus is well documented, there are few data concerning the risk for specific malformations. No statistically significant differences were found among infants of mothers with gestational diabetes mellitus who did not require insulin during pregnancy. Insulin dependent diabetes mellitus is potential risk factor for malformations of central nervous system [34]. Women who experience stressful life events around the time of conception or early gestation may be at increased risk of delivering infants with certain congenital anomalies. For example, in Mexican population in the United States, the occurrence of stressful life events was associated with the risk of neural tube defects. These findings suggest that stress may increase risk in populations with poor nutritional status and poor economic resources [35, 36]. It is likely that not all malformations of the human fetus associated with valproate exposure during pregnancy have a comparable quantitative dose relationship. The reducing of the valproate dose in early pregnancy will provide more effective protection against the spina bifida and other types of fetal malformations [37]. Lupo et al. found an association between environmental level of benzene and the spina bifida. Mothers living in census tracts with the highest benzene levels were more likely to have offspring with the spina bifida than women living in census tracts with the lowest levels [38]. Waller et al. report moderate positive association of maternal obesity with 7 of 16 categories of birth defects. The mechanisms underlying these associations are not yet understood but may be related to undiagnosed diabetes mellitus [39]. Severe obesity has been associated with larger risks of the spina bifida incidence. Underlying mechanisms that have been suggested including aberrant glucose control, oxidative stress, and metabolic syndrome [40]. Higher water nitrate intake was associated with several birth defects in offspring but did not strengthen associations between nitrosatable drugs and birth defects [41]. Cordier et al. report the association between exposure to glycol ethers and neural tube defects, multiple anomalies, and cleft lip [42]. Pesticide exposures were associated with risk of neural tube defects, especially use of pesticides at home and a peri-conceptional residence within 0.25 mile of cultivated fields [43]. Persistent organic pollutants have been associated with a wide range of adverse health effects. Elevated placental concentrations of polycyclic aromatic hydrocarbons, dichlorodiphenyltrichloroethane isomers, and α-hexachloro-cyclohexane are associated with increased risks of neural tube defects [44].

Considerable evidence points to a major genetic component in the spina bifida causation, raising the question of which genes are implicated. In animal spina bifida models more than 40 genetic strains were detected to be associated with this disorder. In some human patients were detected various genetic alterations of coding regions of planar cell polarity genes pathway and genes encoding folate metabolism. The study of folate and its association with neural tube defects is an ongoing endeavor that has led to numerous studies of different genes involved in the folate metabolism pathway, including the most commonly studied thermolabile C677T mutation in the methylenetetrahydrofolate reductase gene [3, 45, 46]. Most of observed genetic alterations are sporadic (non-syndromic), only less than 10% of cases are syndromic, connected with genetic disorders such as trisomy 13 or 18. Up to date evidence supports a theory of a multi-factorial origin of neural tube defects as a consequence of both, genetic and non-genetic factors [47]. Recent studies of mouse mutant with transformation related protein 53 showed that exencephaly susceptibility depends on the presence of two X chromosomes, not the absence of the Y chromosome. Involvement of genetic factors in etiology is supported by evidence that the risk for siblings of spina bifida patient is 2–5%, representing 20 to 50-fold higher risk compared to the general population prevalence of 1 per 1000. Relatives of 2nd and 3rd line display lower risk compared to 1st line relatives, though still increased compared to standard population risk. Woman who has child with spina bifida has approximately 3% risk for another pregnancy affected by spina bifida, risk arises to 10% after two affected pregnancies. The agreement of neural tube defects is higher in monozygotic and dizygotic twins of the same sex compared to twins of the opposite sex. Female excess among cranial neural tube defects is an epigenetic phenomenon whose molecular investigation will produce insight into the mechanisms underlying neural tube defects [3, 48]. Trisomy 18 is the most commonly associated aneuploidy with open neural tube defects. Other genetic disorders include Meckel-Gruber syndrome, Jarcho-Levin dysplasia, HARD (hydrocephalus, agyria and retinal dysplasia), trisomy 13, PHAVER syndrome (pterygia, heart defects, autosomal recessive inheritance, vertebral defects, ear anomalies and radial defects), VATER syndrome (vertebral anomalies, anal atresia, trachea-esophageal fistula and renal abnormalities), and X-linked neural tube defects among others. A significant number of fetuses with open defects are chromosomally abnormal. Although prenatal chromosome analysis should be considered in all cases, prenatal ultrasound seems effective in identifying those fetuses with an underlying chromosomal abnormality. It is questionable how many genes in the human genome pose a risk of neural tube defects. Studies often draw conflicting conclusions due to limitations in the design of studies that affect the strength of statistical analysis. Association studies and sequencing of the entire exome or genome are a way to identify genes that affect the incidence of human neural tube defects [16, 49, 50]. If a prenatal diagnosis of myelomeningocele is suspected, karyotype and genetic consultation should be obtained. Multidisciplinary approach is necessary to treat and support this malformation which is a huge burden on the patient, family, and the society. The most of suspected etiological factors does not have strong evidence or occur less frequently. This underlines to theory of multifactorial etiology of neural tube defects.

4. Pathophysiology

The development of the normal spinal cord from the second to the sixth week of pregnancy includes gastrulation and primary and secondary neurulation. During the first stage of gastrulation, the endoderm and ectoderm form a bilaminar embryonic disc (**Figure 2**). Cell division and migration lead to the formation of a mesoderm and a trilaminar disk is formed. The interaction of the notochord with the ectoderm creates a neuroectoderm. The beginning of the neural plate is in the midline and then extends in the proximal and caudal directions. The pathological effects during primary neurulation can lead to the spinal dysraphism. Part of the primary neurulation is the formation of nerve folds - the nerve groove. By joining the nerve folds, the nerve plate changes into a neural tube. Closure of the cranial and caudal openings of the neural tube represents the end of the process of primary neurulation (**Figure 3**). Disorder of the closure of the caudal neural tube causes the formation of a plaque (exposed nerve tissue). The existence of a neural plaque is a differential feature between myelocele and myelomeningocele [51]. Pluripotent cells forming the caudal end, forms vacuoles and neurons. Their cavitation leads to the formation of a central canal. Apoptosis of said cells leads to the formation of the conus medullaris, filum terminale and ventriculus terminalis. The final closure of the caudal neuropore leads to the transformation from the primary neurulation to the secondary neurulation. During secondary neurulation, the ectoderm and part of the endoderm forms the medullary cord. Two types of cells develop from the medullary epithelium - neuroblasts and spongioblasts. Neuroblasts differentiate

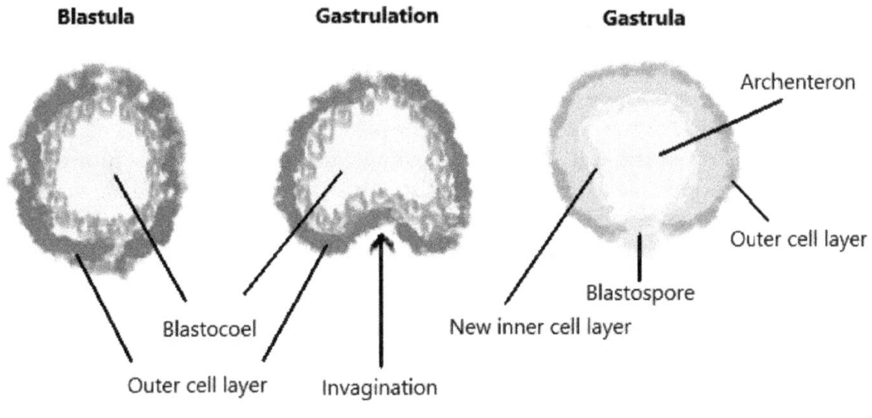

Figure 2.
The process of the gastrulation (author's archive).

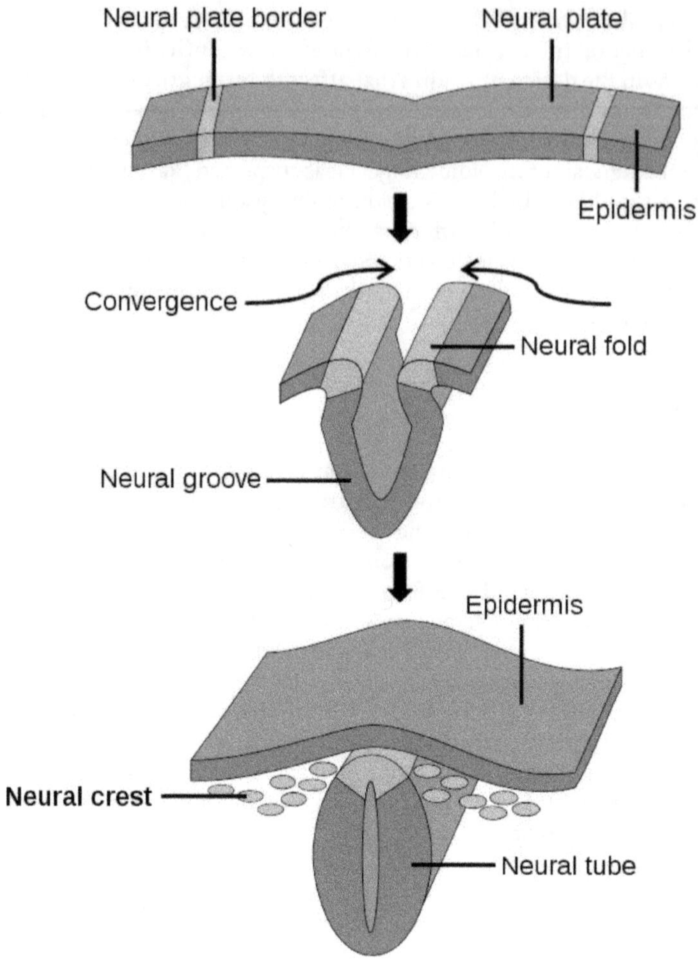

Figure 3.
The process of primary neurulation (public domain, source: wikipedia.org).

into different types of neurons. Ependymal cells, astrocytes and oligodendrocytes differentiate from spongioblasts. The wall of the occluding medullary tube is formed by a layer of cylindrical pluripotent neuroepithelial cells. Towards the cavity, the cells are interconnected by connecting complexes. The luminal surface of the neuroepithelium forms the inner border membrane. From the environment, the neuroepithelium is bounded by a basement membrane, which forms the outer border membrane. As the cells proliferate, the medullary tube wall thickens, making the neuroepithelium multilayered cylindrical. In the area of the future spinal cord, it is possible to histologically distinguish the inner ventricular zone (the primitive ependymal layer), the middle intermediate zone (the future gray matter) and the outer marginal zone (the future white matter). The primitive medullary tube has a thin wall and a wide lumen. Later, the wall is roughened and the lumen has the shape of a slit in cross-section oriented ventrodorsally (the future central canal). On both sides, the cavity is inserted into the wall in the form of a longitudinal notch - sulcus limitans. This incision divides the lateral walls of the neural tube into ventral basal and dorsal alar plate. Neuroblasts of the basal plate become motor neurons, whereas sensory neurons form in the alar plate. In the future spinal cord, unlike the lateral walls, the dorsal and ventral walls do not participate in active cell proliferation. The cells of these parts are mainly involved in the formation of ependyma. The medullary cord separates, gradually condenses and is subject to cavitation. The cavitation combines to form a single tube. The disorder of secondary neurulation is mostly limited to the spinal cord and conditions the formation of closed neural tube defects (neural tissue is not exposed). Factors playing role in etiology of spina bifida, such as genetic, environmental and nutritional factors have mostly effect on neurulation causing its disruption, preventing closure of neuropores and neural folding. Effect of etiological insults is different, disrupting various phases of neural tube formation, but the result in all factors is alike, causing abnormal neurulation [8]. The essential step in pathogenesis of spina bifida is non-union of dorsal spinal structures, in severe forms it is failure of embryonic neural tube closure. Immature neural tube remains uncovered or is covered only by a thin membrane what causes direct exposure of the developing and open neural tube to the amniotic fluid. After relatively normal initial development, neuronal differentiation of bifid neuroepithelium and development of spinal motor and sensitive functions in whole extent including levels below the lesion, with the progression of gestation, destructive effect of exposure of the developing spinal cord to the amniotic fluid manifests as necrosis of neurons and micro-hemorrhagic changes of the spinal cord [3]. Pathological examination of the spinal cords of stillborn human fetuses with myelomeningocele demonstrate varying degrees of neural tissue loss at the site of the defect, but normal-appearing dorsal and ventral horns proximal of the lesion. Recently produced experimental evidence suggests that secondary traumatic injury and degenerative changes, acquired in utero, to the openly exposed neural tissue may be primarily responsible for the massive neurological deficit associated with myelomeningocele. In myelomeningocele as the severe degree of spina bifida the defect consists of dorsally opened vertebral arch, as well as dorsal defect of dura mater that is laterally attached to the dermal layer and defect in layer of pia mater which is fused to the epidermis. The unclosed spinal cord is directly exposed without any covering to the amniotic fluid and later to the surrounding environment. On the surface of spinal cord is only membrane - the abnormal arachnoid sac – which is unable of providing protection against traumatic injury caused by toxic exposition. Another insult to the nervous tissue can occur during passage through the birth canal in case of vaginal delivery leading to further hemorrhage and abrasion. The devastating role of secondary insult to the exposed nervous tissue underlines the presence of dorsal and ventral parts of the spinal cord with developed nerve roots and ganglia, what is evidence of preexisting appropriate early embryogenic development. This finding emphasizes the role of early in utero surgery in protection from secondary injury caused by prolonged exposition of the unprotected neural tissue to the amniotic fluid and in preservation of neurological functions [52, 53]. Regular sonographic observations of human fetuses with myelomeningocele show progressive deterioration of leg movements during pregnancy [54]. Experimental data on fetuses with the spina bifida aperta strongly indicate that a discrepancy exists between the occurrence of prenatal leg movements and the spinal location of the meningomyelocele on the one hand, and between the occurrence of pre- and postnatal leg movements [55]. In hemimyelocele, half of the dysgraphic spinal cord is not covered by the dura mater and is exposed to the intrauterine environment. The correlating lower limb shows a motor or sensitive deficit, while the function of the other lower limb is normal or only slightly altered [56]. Staged series of animal fetuses with myelomeningocele have demonstrated gain of neurological function even after the lesion has formed, followed by loss of this function. This finding correlates with a progressive loss of spinal cord tissue integrity. Stiefel et al. studied the development of neuronal connections and neurological function of mice during fetal and neonatal stages in a genetic model of exposed lumbosacral spina bifida. Their findings support the hypothesis that neurological deficits in human myelomeningocele arise after secondary destruction of nerve tissue and loss of function during pregnancy [57]. Meuli et al. report findings that secondary neural tissue destruction during pregnancy is primarily responsible for the functional loss and that timely in utero repair of the open spina bifida might rescue neurologic function [58]. Drewek et al. dealt with the toxic effects of human amniotic fluid on organotypic cultures of rat spinal cord. Using a lactate dehydrogenase outflow test to evaluate toxicity, amniotic fluid was found to become toxic at approximately 34 weeks of gestation. This toxic effect of amniotic fluid occurs relatively suddenly. Surgical closure of a myelomeningocele defect prior to the onset of amniotic fluid toxicity has the potential to prevent injury to sensitive myelodysplastic spinal cord tissue [59].

4.1 Genetic factors

The number of mouse mutants and strains with neural tube defects at present exceeds 240, including 205 representing specific genes, 30 for unidentified genes, and 9 multifactorial strains. Some mutations in isolation do not cause neural tube disorders, but are caused by di-genic, tri-genic, and oligo-genic combinations. This fact corresponds to the nature of the genetic etiology of human neural tube defects. Experimental mouse mutants that have only exencephaly are 4-fold more frequent than those that have spina bifida aperta with or without exencephaly. Many diverse cellular functions and biochemical pathways are involved; the mutants with neural tube defect draw new attention to chromatin modification, the protease-activated receptor cascade, and the ciliopathies. Few mutants directly involve folate metabolism. The research of many mutants is the basis for a complete understanding of the processes of elevation and fusion of nerve folds along mechanically distinct cranial-caudal segments of the neural tube [60]. Neural tube closure is affected by many cellular biological functions, with cytoskeletal, cell cycle, and molecular regulation of cell viability present in mutant mice. Neural tube closure is also affected by transcriptional regulators and proteins that affect chromatin structure. Folic acid supplementation is one of the most effective methods of primary prevention of some neural tube disorders in humans, although the mechanism of action of folate is unclear. In cases where folic acid has no preventive effect, it is possible to reduce the risk of mouse mutants by administering inositol. This finding may determine the strategy for preventing neural tube defects in the future [61]. Exencephaly, the developmental precursor of anencephaly, is most commonly encountered after gene mutation in mice, but spina bifida aperta is also observed in more than 40 mutant strains. Rare putative mutations in the planar cell polarity genes Vangl2 (Vang-like protein 2), Scrib (Scribble planar cell polarity protein), Dact1 (Disheveled binding antagonist of β-catenin 1), and Celsr1 (Cadherin EGF LAG seven-pass G-type receptor 1) cumulatively contribute to over 20% of cases with craniorachischisis, a rare defect; no contributing variants were found for Prickle1 (Prickle planar cell polarity protein 1) or Ptk7 (Protein tyrosine kinase 7). Planar cell polarity rare putative mutations have a weaker role in myelomeningocele, being found in approximately 6% of cases and cumulated across Celsr1, Fuz (Fuzzy planar cell polarity protein), Fzd6 (Frizzled class receptor 6), Prickle1, Vangl1 (Vang-like protein 1), and Vangl2. These results demonstrate that planar cell polarity - gene alterations contribute to the etiology of human neural tube defects [60, 62]. Opposite to unaffected individuals, patients with neural tube defects display though rare, but present missense gene mutations were confirmed by sequenation of the coding regions of human orthologues of these genes. Substantial part of neural tube defects is associated with variants in genes of the planar cell polarity and a non-canonical Wnt signaling pathways [62]. This is particularly significant, since planar cell polarity-gene mutations are potent causes of mouse neural tube defects, generating several phenotypes particularly the severe defect craniorachischisis. Initiation of neural tube closure is disrupted in homozygous mice due to the presence of mutations in planar cell polarity genes. This fact provides a strong association between neural tube defects and planar cell polarity signaling. Missense gene sequence variants detected in humans with neural tube defects are heterozygous and have a wider range of phenotypes than in mouse mutants. It is the interactions between mutations in several heterozygous genes that may be responsible for neural tube defects in humans [63]. Genes of folate one-carbon metabolism are another group of genes linked to neural tube defects. Methylene tetrahydrofolate reductase is an enzyme essential for conversion of homocysteine to methionine generating 5-methyltetrahydrofolate. Variant of this gene 677C > T results in the conversion of valine to alanine at codon 222. This variant causes reduced activity of this enzyme. The homozygous 677TT genotype, in either mother or fetus, particularly in connection with folate deficiency could be a risk factor for neural tube defects. The examination of non-Latin European studies revealed that the association of homozygous dominant genotype with neural tube defect has only been proven for Irish populations, both by case–control studies, and by family-based tests, such as the allele transmission disequilibrium test [64]. Pickell et al. refer that biological evidence linking maternal methylene-tetrahydrofolate reductase and folate deficiencies to adverse pregnancy outcomes in mice mutants. It underscores the importance of folate in reducing the incidence of early embryonic defects and in the prevention of the development of placental abnormalities that may increase susceptibility to other defects [65]. The glycine cleavage system is a multi-enzyme component of mitochondrial folate metabolism, and glycine cleavage system-encoding genes therefore represent candidates for involvement in neural tube defects. Mutations in genes of the glycine cleavage system, which reduce the activity of two mitochondrial enzymes of folate-mediated one-carbon metabolism (glycine-decarboxylase and amino-methyltransferase), are also found among patients with neural tube defects and in this case loss of function of the mouse orthologues produces neural tube defects [66]. Glycine decarboxylase in the glycine cleavage system acts to transfer one carbon unit to the folate metabolism of one carbon. Mutations in glycine decarboxylase cause a rare recessive disease - non-ketotic hyperglycemia. However, these mutations have also been identified in patients with neural tube disorders. Nevertheless, the relationship between non-ketotic hyperglycemia and neural tube disorders remains unclear. Formate supplementation normalizes the folate profile, restores embryonic growth and prevents neural tube defects, suggesting that glycine decarboxylase-deficiency causes neural tube defects through limiting supply of one-carbon units from mitochondrial folate metabolism [67]. Mitochondrial enzyme activity supplies 70% of the cell's one-carbon units for metabolism, as formate molecules, and it seems possible that genetic variants in this pathway may prove to be important risk factors for neural tube defects [3].

4.2 Non-genetic factors

A variety of environmental factors have been linked with neural tube defects (**Table 1**). Folic acid seems to play crucial role in the pathophysiology of neural tube disorders. It is inevitable in the synthesis of deoxyribonucleic acid and ribonucleic acid precursors. Dihydrofolate reductases convert folic acid into tetrahydrofolate. Essential step is methylation of the folic acid that is responsible for its functionality. Supplementation of folic acid is linked with decreased incidence of neural tube defects by 71% [68]. Animal studies have not provided enough information to establish metabolic and genomic mechanism underlying human folic acid responsiveness in neural tube defects [69]. 5-methyl-tetrahydrofolate is the active co-factor of enzymes involving one-carbon transfer reactions forming purine and pyrimidine. Folate receptors take up MTHF into the cell, glutamates and carrier protein can be added to form polyglutamate folates that cannot cross cell membranes. Folic acid is directly associated with cell proliferation as for in neurulation. Neural folds express the folate receptors. The absence of folic acid halts neural tissue proliferation and migration during neurulation leading to neural tube disorders. In the last decades there has been significant worldwide decrease in overall incidence of neural tube defects due to the periconceptional supplementation of folic acid. Folate food fortification became priority in many countries. However, despite indisputable benefits of folic acid supplementation neural tube defects continue to be a substantial part of perinatal morbidity and mortality worldwide. Recent studies demonstrating novel roles and interactions between innate immune factors such as the complement cascade, neurulation, and folate metabolism are explored [70]. Despite the great effect of the folate food fortification programs, there are still cases of neural tube defects also after periconceptional supplementation. This might be due to defects in folate metabolism, receptors or transport proteins that put these women into higher susceptibility. Genetic alterations leading to impaired structure or function of receptor proteins, particularly α- and β-folate-receptors, which have function in neural cells, can lead to failure in neurulation [8, 71]. The C677T polymorphism in the methylenetetrahydrofolate reductase gene has been reported to play a critical role in the pathogenesis of neural tube defects. This association has been widely demonstrated, but the results are inconclusive. Meta-analysis performed to rule out the relation between C677T polymorphism in the methylenetetrahydrofolate reductase gene and neural tube defects demonstrated that this mutation decreases the activity of enzymes required for folate metabolism, thus reducing the serum folate concentration. Yang et al. found no association between any of the fathers' genotypes and neural tube defects, whereas a significant correlation between C677T polymorphism in the methylene-tetrahydrofolate reductase gene and neural tube defect-risk was found in patients with neural tube defect and in their mother [8, 72]. Folate antagonists such as phenytoin, valproic acid, and carbamazepine have a direct effect on neural tube defects due to inhibiting the activity of folate [73]. Apoptosis and proliferation play important roles in embryonic development and are required for neural tube closure. The antifolate drug methotrexate induces folate dysmetabolism by inhibition of dihydrofolate reductase and causes abnormal apoptosis and proliferation. Methotrexate causes a folate and folate-associated dysmetabolism, and further induced abnormal apoptosis and proliferation, which may play a critical role in the occurrence of neural tube defects caused by folate deficiency [74]. Mutation in homeobox genes and fibroblast growth factor dysfunction has some roles in the pathogenesis of neural tube defects [8]. The important role of vitamin B12 in development of nervous system is known. It is necessary in folate metabolism in converting homocysteine from this metabolic pathway into methionine. Along with methionine synthase it reduces the toxicity of homocysteine. Under circumstances of vitamin B12 deficiency homocysteine serum levels increase. The high homocysteine level can cause posttranslational modification of folate receptors that can after modification represent an autoantigen. Production of antibodies against these autoantigens leads to decrease of folate activity [8, 70]. Valproic acid is widely used to treat epilepsy and bipolar disorder and is also a potent teratogen, but its mechanisms of action in any of these settings are unknown. This anticonvulsant increases risk of neural tube defects by 10-fold when taken during the first trimester of pregnancy [67]. Potent histone deacetylase inhibitory activity of valproic acid may disturb the balance of protein acetylation and deacetylation, leading to neurulation failure [75]. Valproic acid activates transcription from diverse exogenous and endogenous promoters and have teratogenic effects in vertebrate embryos, while non-teratogenic analogues of valproic acid do not inhibit histone deacetylase and do not activate transcription [76]. Production of neural tube defects due to fumonisin (group of mycotoxins derived from Fusarium and their Liseola section) exposure in rodent embryos has identified sphingosine phosphate metabolism as a key target of the toxin, potentially compromising folate utilization [3]. Neural tube defects are among the most common of the malformations associated with diabetic embryopathy. Pax3 (paired box 3) is an important developmental control gene, the expression of which is impaired in the embryos of diabetic mice, and therefore neural tube apoptosis occurs [77].

4.3 Pathogenesis of open spinal dysraphism

Two phases of neural tube formation occur in higher vertebrates: closure and canalization. Primary neurulation is initiated at the boundary between future hindbrain and cervical spine on day 22 after fertilization (**Figure 3**). At the rostral extremity of the forebrain begins closure and backwards continues zipping to meet forward closure from the hindbrain. On the 24th postconceptional day rostral neuropore closure is completed, spinal closure lasts longer till the 26th day, progressively forming lower parts of the neuroaxis. Meningomyelocele is an open defect of neural tube as a result of closure failure of the neural folds in the dorsal midline. It can be consequence of failure of any part of neurulation process. Craniorachischisis is the most severe neural tube defect with almost completely dorsally opened brain and spine. This defect is a result of closure failure on 22nd day. Analysis of mice with mutations of Vangl2 gene has revealed a defect of late gastrulation. The process of convergent extension involves the intercalation of cells in the midline to lengthen and narrow the body axis [3]. Planar cell polarity signaling is necessary for initiation of neural tube closure in higher vertebrates. In mice with planar cell polarity gene mutations, a broad embryonic midline prevents the onset of neurulation through wide spacing of the neural folds. Cellular autonomic error of convergent spread requiring planar cell polarity signaling via Rho-associated protein kinase plays a role in development of neural tube defects [78]. Anencephaly is a defect of neural tube closure where initial closure is successful but cranial neurulation fails. Open spina bifida defects are results of failure in subsequent spinal neurulation. These lesions can be of various levels and sizes depending on the stage at which the 'zipping' process fails [3]. The molecular mechanism based on the antagonism of Bmp2 (Bone morphogenetic protein 2) signaling is the basis for the regulation of the formation of dorsolateral hinge points during mouse neural tube closure. Spinal closure in the curly tail (Grainy head like transcription factor 3) mutant fails later, due to enhanced curvature of the body axis, producing a spina bifida confined to the lumbar and sacral region [79]. Zic2-mutant (Zic family member 2) mice fail early in spinal neurulation, owing to lack of dorsolateral neural plate bending, and display a large spina bifida from thoracic level downwards [78].

4.4 Pathogenesis of closed spinal dysraphism

Secondary neurulation is responsible for forming of the neural tube in the low sacro-coccygeal regions, following the closure of the caudal neuropore. The end of the embryo comprises the tail bud whose mesenchymal cell core progressively reorganizes into longitudinal cell condensations. The most dorsal of these condensations undergoes canalization, converting the solid neural precursor into epithelial secondary neural tube [77, 80]. Closed spinal dysraphisms are covered with skin and they are not in contact with surrounding environment as they are consequence of failure of secondary neurulation. Occult spina bifida is outcome of inappropriate separation and differentiation of neural and mesenchymal tissues. Research helped to identify a bipotential neuro-mesodermal precursor cell lineage within the tail bud. Differentiation and separation of these precursor cells are essential for proper development and existence of this cells explains incomplete separation of these layers in case of its malfunction. The histological and ultrastructural properties of secondary neurulation in C57BL/6 mouse embryos were examined as a first step to analyze the cause of the presence of this process in mammalian embryos. Secondary neurulation in mouse embryos consists of two phases - platelet formation and cavitation. These two events occur simultaneously. The medullary rosette consists of elongated tail bud cells, radially arranged around a central lumen formed by cavitation. The secondary portion of the neural tube forms in 10-day embryos by progressive enlargement of the central lumen and addition of tail bud cells to the rosette. The medullary plate also consists of elongated tail bud cells. These cells expand ventrally from the basal aspect of the dorsal superficial ectoderm into the slit-like cavity formed by cavitation. The formation of the secondary neural tube occurs in 11- to 12-day-old embryos in the process of forming additional lateral and ventral tail cells into the medullary plate. Free cells and cell debris that do not show signs of necrosis often occur in the forming lumen of the secondary neural tube. Small intercellular junctions form at the juxta-luminal ends of the tail bud cells during the formation of the medullary rosette or plate, and cavitation occurs. Cavitation per se during secondary neurulation is a relatively passive phenomenon, which results principally from neighboring cells becoming polarized apicobasal and incorporated into a primitive neuroepithelium. The latter constitutes the walls of the forming secondary neural tube [3, 81]. The clinical observation that the distal spinal cord is often tethered to surrounding tissues, in spina bifida occulta, can therefore be recognized as a disorder of secondary neurulation. The frequent and striking association of closed spinal dysraphism with intradural lipoma is not well explained. The progressive generation of axial tissues (spinal cord, skeleton and musculature) of the body has long been proposed to depend on the activity of multipotent stem cells. The data strongly support their existence, there is little definitive information about their multipotency or extent of contribution to the axis [3, 82]. Spinal lipomas are the most common form of occult spinal dysraphism. Lipomas represent a wide spectrum of diseases in regard to pathological anatomy, symptomatology, and treatment options. These lesions are united by a similar embryology and pathophysiology. The treatment of these lesions is controversial. Some physicians advocating surgical treatment for all patients regardless of clinical symptoms and others proposing that surgery in cases of the clinical manifestation [83].

4.5 Postnatal pathogenesis of the spina bifida

The spina bifida is associated with another brain malformations and development of the hydrocephalus. Brain defects involve the spectrum of anomalies related to the Chiari II malformation in about 90% of cases [83]. Chiari II malformation is associated with herniation of normal-sized cerebellum caudally through the foramen magnum [84]. Insufficient distribution of the embryonic ventricular system can be considered to be the cause of Chiari II malformation in children with myelomeningocele. Defective occlusion and an open neural tube secrete fluid accumulation, which affects the normal development of the brain. These mechanisms result in small posterior fossa and disorganization of the brain [85]. Volume reduction of the cerebellum is more associated with thoracic level spinal lesions than lumbar or sacral lesions. Few volumetric MRI studies of the entire cerebellum have been published. Even less quantitative information is available in patients with hindbrain malformations, including the Chiari II malformation which is ubiquitous in patients with meningomyelocele. Children with thoracic level lesions have smaller cerebellar volumes relative to those with lumbo-sacral lesions, who had smaller volumes compared to children without the pathological development. The reduction in cerebellar volume in children with meningomyelocele represents a reconfiguration involving anterior lobe enlargement and posterior lobe reduction [86]. Most of patients with open spinal defect display abnormal MRI finding. Distortion of the midbrain where colliculi fuse into a single beak pointing posteriorly and invaginate into cerebellum are present in about 65% of cases [3]. About 70% of patients have elongated medulla with kinking at the spino-medullary junction [83]. The basal ganglia and subcortical structures usually have normal appearance on MRI. Meningomyelocele differentially disrupts brain regions whereby some structures are volumetrically normal whereas others are reduced or enlarged. In hippocampus, volumetric reduction coupled with increased mean diffusivity may imply reduce cellular density and aberrant organization. The increased volume and markedly reduced mean diffusivity of putamen indicate increased density. The hippocampus, but not the amygdala, is reduced in volume, and the putamen is enlarged [3, 87]. Almost half of the children with meningomyelocele have hypogenesis of the corpus callosum involving either the splenium and posterior body or the rostrum [83]. The results of the Treble-Barna et al. study contribute to emerging evidence of memory impairment in adults with meningomyelocele and provide quantitative evidence of impaired hippocampal macrostructure as a neural correlate of memory impairment in this population. These anomalies suggest that the disruption of neural migration associated with meningomyelocele is prolonged into the second trimester, since the corpus callosum develops from 8 to 20 weeks prenatally [88]. Anomalies of the corpus callosum are an important indicator of additional brain anomalies. Quantitative studies show marked volume and integrity differences, especially posteriorly in cases with hypogenesis or severe hypoplasia [89]. The hypoplastic corpus callosum is not macro- or microstructurally intact in cases of the spina bifida, even when it appears radiologically intact. Both volume and integrity of posterior regions are related to reductions in intelligence quotient and to interhemispheric processing. Reduced integrity of the corpus callosum has been shown also in the genu, but not in commissura anterior [90]. Anomalies of the corpus callosum are associated with reduced interhemispheric communication and general difficulties integrating information in language, reading, and social domains [3]. Abnormalities of the corpus callosum are known to occur in the majority of patients with Chiari II malformation, and also callosal defects can be associated with spinal closed dysraphism. Chiari II malformation is associated with eye movement difficulties as well as problems with the precision and timing of motor movements and rhythmicity. When the neuroaxis emerges as a whole, the structures of embryological ectodermal origin and cranial and spinal structures are not independent regions from each other and thus, asymptomatic closed spinal dysraphisms have been demonstrated to accompany dysgenesis of the corpus callosum [91]. Secondary consequences of the spina bifida include hydrocephalus which results primarily from obstruction of cerebrospinal fluid flow at the IV. ventricle level, with other factors including aqueductal stenosis, venous hemodynamics and ependymal denudation. Cortical reorganization occurs around the area of ventricular dilatation [3]. Frontal regions are enlarged and there is a reduction in the volume of posterior cortical regions [92]. The reduction of cortex thickness and also white matter is associated with the mechanical effects of hydrocephalus. Overall reduction in white matter and increased neocortical thickness in the frontal lobes suggest that the spina bifida reflects a long-term disruption of brain development that extends far beyond the neural tube defect [93]. Hydrocephalus associated with the spina bifida is caused by an obstruction of the cerebrospinal fluid flow from IV. ventricular or malformation of the cerebral aqueduct. Ventriculomegaly causes systematic destruction of white matter periventricular axons. Motor, sensory, visual as well as memory systems can be disrupted by stiffening of periventricular structures, including the corpus callosum and the fimbria-fornix pathway. Secondary changes occur in neuronal cell bodies and synapses, with neurons not undergoing apoptosis. The clinical syndrome of hydrocephalic brain dysfunction is caused by subcortical detachment. Some of the brain dysfunctions are reversible due to the restoration of blood flow through the brain and the normalization of the extracellular environment [94]. Diffusion tensor tractography revealed diffusion tensor characteristics of myelination impairment and pathological development as well as abnormalities in intrinsic axonal characteristics and extra-axonal space in the association pathways of children with the development of the spina bifida. The differences in the diffusion metrics are suggestive of the pathological white matter development and persistent degeneration with increased age [95]. Hydrocephalus exerts primarily a linear effect on cognitive and motor outcomes. Deviations from normative standards for volumes of frontal versus posterior regions are associated with reductions in intelligence quotient and fine motor dexterity [3]. With the exception of fine motor skills and small differences in memory and spatial domains, children with spina bifida and arrested or shunt-dependent hydrocephalus have similar neuropsychological profiles [96]. Patients with the spina bifida have extensive motor deficits in the trunk, upper limbs, eyes, and speech articulators that correspond to disorders characteristic for cerebellar lesions. The structure and function of the brain correlates with a number of motor dysfunctions. Motor learning is maintained in the spina bifida. Pathological are motor functions that require predictive signals and accurate calibration of motion time signs. This creates a deficit in the coordination of smooth movement and the cerebellar triad - ataxia, dysmetria, and dysarthria. Said motor function in individuals with the spina bifida is impaired phenotypically very similarly to cerebellar lesions. The age-based cerebellar motor plasticity is limited in individuals with this neurodevelopmental disorder [97]. Attention deficit reflecting problems with posterior attention systems involving orienting and arousal mediated by the midbrain, with tectal anomalies directly correlated with the severity of difficulties with stimulus control. Procedural learning and attention functions involving sustained attention and persistence are relatively preserved, possibly reflecting less impairment in frontal-striatal regions and basal ganglia [3, 98]. Impairments in attentional disengagement in the spina bifida are not attributable to the general effects of hydrocephalus but are instead associated with specific midbrain anomalies that are part of the Chiari II malformation [99]. Development of individuals with severe forms of spina bifida throughout the lifetime is strongly affected by neurocognitive and movement disorders. Neurocognitive difficulties cause problems in keeping attention, learning, language comprehension and pragmatics as well as in assimilation of information. Procedural learning, word reading, vocabulary and social activation are usually not affected. Infants with spina bifida do not learn motor contingencies as easily or at the same rate as infants with typical development and are more likely to decrease motor responses when sensory feedback is absent. Intellectual disability is relatively infrequent, affecting perhaps 20–25% of people with the spina bifida and often after complications associated with the hydrocephalus. Status of cognitive functions in spina bifida patients is very variable as well as intelligence quotient scores. Impairment of intelligence and cognitive skills is mostly associated with presence of possible complications, such as hydrocephalus. Treatment of hydrocephalus is burdened with eventual complications as shunt obstruction, malfunction or infections. Repeated shunt complications can have impact on intellectual performance. Environmental and socio-economic factors also influence achieved abilities. Motor and cognitive outcomes are directly related to level and extent of spinal lesion, what reflects the association of more severe brain pathology with higher level and bigger extent of defect [3, 100]. Executive function impairments potentially have a detrimental effect on the individual's emotional health and coping. Goal management training is a cognitive rehabilitation method for improving executive function. Compensatory intervention to manage executive dysfunction, effective and lasting benefits can be achieved in regard to aspects of perceived emotional health and coping [101].

5. Conclusion

The spina bifida involves congenital problems that result in abnormal bone formation in the spine and spinal cord. Closed spinal dysraphism is the mildest form of the neural tube defects which involves a hidden vertebral defect and minimal neural involvement. Open spinal dysraphism refers to a defect in which neural tissues communicate with the external environment such as meningocele and myelomeningocele. The incidence of neural tube defects has different rates among different ethnicity, geography, gender, and also countries. Various nutritional, maternal and environmental factors play a role in the etiology and pathogenesis of the spina bifida. However, the impact of these factors is ambiguous and further research is needed in this area.

Conflict of interest

The authors declare no conflict of interest.

Appendices and Nomenclature

T – thoracic vertebra.
L – lumbar vertebra.
WHO – World Health Organization.
EUROCAT – European network of population-based registries for the epidemiological surveillance of congenital anomalies.
C677T – variant of methylenetetrahydrofolate reductase.
Vangl1 – Vang-like protein 1.
Vangl2 – Vang-like protein 2.
Scrib – Scribble planar cell polarity protein.
Dact1 – Disheveled binding antagonist of β-catein 1.
Celsr1 – Cadherin EGF LAG seven-pass G-type receptor 1.
Prickle1 – Prickle planar cell polarity protein 1.
Ptk7 – Protein tyrosine kinase 7.
Fuz – Fuzzy planar cell polarity protein.
Fzd6 – Frizzled class receptor 7.
Pax3 – Paired box 3.
Bmp2 – Bone morphogenetic protein 2.
Zic2 – Zic family member 2.
C57BL/6 – inbred strain of laborytory mouse.
MRI – magnetic resonance imaging.

Author details

René Opšenák*, Romana Richterová and Branislav Kolarovszki
Jessenius Faculty of Medicine in Martin, Comenius University in Bratislava, University Hospital Martin, Martin, Slovakia

*Address all correspondence to: opsenak@gmail.com

References

[1] Venkataramana NK. Spinal dysraphism. J Pediatr Neurosci. 2011;6(Suppl 1):31-40.

[2] Iftikhar W, De Jesus O. Spinal Dysraphism And Myelomeningocele. In: StatPearls. Treasure Island (FL): StatPearls Publishing; August 10, 2020.

[3] Copp AJ el al. Spina bifida. Nat Rev Dis Primers. 2015;1:15007.

[4] Oakeshott P et al. Open spina bifida: birth findings predict long-term outcome. Arch Dis Child. 2012;97:474-476.

[5] Yi Y et al. Economic burden of neural tube defects and impact of prevention with folic acid: a literature review. Eur J Pediatr. 2011;170:1391-1400

[6] Sahmat A et al. The Prevalence and Distribution of Spina Bifida in a Single Major Referral Center in Malaysia. Front Pediatr. 2017;5:237.

[7] Windham GC et al. The association of twinning and neural tube defects: studies in Los Angeles, California, and Norway. Acta Genet Med Gemellol (Roma). 1982;31(3-4):165-172.

[8] Bhandari J, Thada PK. Neural Tube Disorders. In: StatPearls. Treasure Island (FL): StatPearls Publishing; April 13, 2020.

[9] Zaganjor I et al. Describing the Prevalence of Neural Tube Defects Worldwide: A Systematic Literature Review. PLoS ONE. 2016;11(4):151-586.

[10] Bauer SB et al. Urodynamic evaluation of boy with myelodysplasia and incontinence. Urology. 1977;10(4):354-362.

[11] Mehrotra A et al. Cervicothoracic Spinal Dysraphism: Unravelling the Pandora's Box. J Pediatr Neurosci. 2019;14(4):203-210.

[12] Netto JM et al. Spinal dysraphism: a neurosurgical review for the urologist. Rev Urol. 2009;11(2):71-81.

[13] Trudell AS, Odibo AO. Diagnosis of spina bifida on ultrasound: always termination? Best Pract Res Clin Obstet Gynaecol. 2014;28(3):367-377.

[14] Liu J et al. The recurrence risk of neural tube defects (NTDs) in a population with high prevalence of NTDs in northern China. Oncotarget. 2017;8(42):72577-72583.

[15] Sebold CD et al. Recurrence risks for neural tube defects in siblings of patients with lipomyelomeningocele. Genet. Med. 2005;7(1):64-67.

[16] Sahni M, Ohri A. StatPearls [Internet]. StatPearls Publishing; Treasure Island (FL): Mar 24, 2020. Meningomyelocele.

[17] Atta CA et al. Global birth prevalence of spina bifida by folic acid fortification status: a systematic review and meta-analysis. Am J Public Health. 2016;106:24-34.

[18] Blencowe H et al. Estimates of global and regional prevalence of neural tube defects for 2015: a systematic analysis. Ann N Y Acad Sci. 2018;1414:31-46.

[19] Bodin CR et al. Ultrasound in Prenatal Diagnostics and Its Impact on the Epidemiology of Spina Bifida in a National Cohort from Denmark with a Comparison to Sweden. Biomed Res Int. 2018;2018:9203-9985.

[20] Velie EM, Shaw GM. Impact of prenatal diagnosis and elective termination on prevalence and risk estimates of neural tube defects in California, 1989-1991. Am J Epidemiol. 1996;144:473-479.

[21] Dolk H et al. The prevalence of congenital anomalies in Europe. Adv Exp Med Biol. 2010;686:349-364.

[22] Avagliano L et al. Cell death and cell proliferation in human spina bifida. Birth Defects Res. Part A Clin. Mol. Teratol. 2016;106(2):104-113.

[23] Grewal J et al. Maternal periconceptional smoking and alcohol consumption and risk for select congenital anomalies. Birth Defects Res A Clin Mol Teratol. 2008;82:519-526.

[24] Schmidt RJ et al. Maternal caffeine consumption and risk of neural tube defects. Birth Defects Res A Clin Mol Teratol. 2009;85:879-889.

[25] Kirke PN et al. Maternal plasma folate and vitamin B12 are independent risk factors for neural tube defects. Q J Med. 1993;86:703-708.

[26] Carmichael SL et al. Reduced risks of neural tube defects and orofacial clefts with higher diet quality. Arch Pediatr Adolesc Med. 2012;166:121-126.

[27] Yazdy MM et al. Maternal dietary glycaemic intake during pregnancy and the risk of birth defects. Paediatr Perinat Epidemiol. 2011;25:340-346.

[28] Shaw GM et al. Is dietary intake of methionine associated with a reduction in risk for neural tube defect-affected pregnancies. Teratology. 1997;56:295-299.

[29] Shaw GM et al. Choline and risk of neural tube defects in a folate-fortified population. Epidemiology. 2009;20:714-719.

[30] Ray JG, Blom HJ. Vitamin B12 insufficiency and the risk of fetal neural tube defects. Q J Med. 2003;96:289-295.

[31] Velie EM et al. Maternal supplemental and dietary zinc intake and the occurrence of neural tube defects in California. Am J Epidemiol. 1999;150:605-616.

[32] Moretti ME et al. Maternal hyperthermia and the risk for neural tube defects in offspring: systematic review and metaanalysis. Epidemiology. 2005;16:216-219.

[33] Wasserman CR et al. Socioeconomic status, neighborhood social conditions, and neural tube defects. Am J Publ Health. 1998;88:1674-1680.

[34] Becerra JE et al. Diabetes mellitus during pregnancy and the risks for specific birth defects: a population-based case-control study. Pediatrics. 1990;85:1-9.

[35] Carmichael SL, Shaw GM. Maternal life event stress and congenital anomalies. Epidemiology. 2000;11:30-35.

[36] Suarez L et al. Maternal stress, social support, and risk of neural tube defects among Mexican Americans. Epidemiology. 2003;14:612-616.

[37] Vajda FJ et al. Dose dependence of fetal malformations associated with valproate. Neurology. 2013;81:999-1003.

[38] Lupo PJ et al. Maternal exposure to ambient levels of benzene and neural tube defects among offspring: Texas, 1999-2004. Environ Health Perspect. 2011;119:397-402.

[39] Waller DK, et al. Prepregnancy obesity as a risk factor for structural birth defects. Arch Pediatr Adolesc Med. 2007;161:745-750.

[40] Carmichael SL et al. Prepregnancy obesity: a complex risk factor for selected birth defects. Birth Defects Res A Clin Mol Teratol. 2010;88:804-810.

[41] Brender JD et al. Prenatal nitrate intake from drinking water and selected birth defects in offspring of participants

in the national birth defects prevention study. Environ Health Perspect. 2013;121:1083-1089.

[42] Cordier S, et al. Congenital malformations and maternal occupational exposure to glycol ethers. Epidemiology. 1997;8:355-363.

[43] Brender JD et al. Maternal pesticide exposure and neural tube defects in Mexican Americans. Ann Epidemiol. 2010;20:16-22.

[44] Ren A et al. Association of selected persistent organic pollutants in the placenta with the risk of neural tube defects. Proc Natl Acad Sci USA. 2011;138:12770-12775.

[45] Alruwaili AA, M Das J. Myelomeningocele. In: StatPearls. Treasure Island (FL): StatPearls Publishing; June 30, 2020.

[46] Northrup H, Volcik KA. Spina bifida and other neural tube defects. Curr Probl Pediatr. 2000;30(10):313-332.

[47] Rampersaud E et al. In: Neural Tube Defects: From Origin to Treatment. Wyszynski DF, editor. Oxford Univ. Press 2006;165-175.

[48] Juriloff DM, Harris MJ. Hypothesis: the female excess in cranial neural tube defects reflects an epigenetic drag of the inactivating X chromosome on the molecular mechanisms of neural fold elevation. Birth Defects Res A Clin Mol Teratol. 2012;94:849-855.

[49] Sepulveda W et al. Chromosomal abnormalities in fetuses with open neural tube defects: prenatal identification with ultrasound. Ultrasound Obstet Gynecol. 2004;23(4):352-356.

[50] Au KS et al. Epidemiologic and genetic aspects of spina bifida and other neural tube defects. Dev Disabil Res Rev. 2010;16(1):6-15.

[51] Alruwaili AA, M Das J. Myelomeningocele. 2020 Oct 13. In: StatPearls [Internet]. Treasure Island (FL): StatPearls Publishing; Jan, 2021.

[52] Meuli M, et al. The spinal cord lesion in human fetuses with myelomeningocele: Implications for fetal surgery. J Pediatr Surg. 1997;32:448-452.

[53] Hutchins GM, et al. Acquired spinal cord injury in human fetuses with myelomeningocele. Pediatr Pathol Lab Med. 1996;16:701-712.

[54] Korenromp MJ et al. Early fetal leg movements in myelo-meningocele. Lancet. 1986;327:917-918.

[55] Sival DA et al. Perinatal motor behaviour and neurological outcome in spina bifida aperta. Early Hum Dev. 1997;50:27-37.

[56] Duckworth T et al. Hemimyelocele. Dev Med Child Neurol. 1968;10:69-75. (Suppl. 16)

[57] Stiefel D et al. Fetal spina bifida: loss of neural function in utero. J Neurosurg. 2007;106:213-221.

[58] Meuli M et al. In utero surgery rescues neurological function at birth in sheep with spina bifida. Nat Med. 1995;1:342-347.

[59] Drewek MJ et al. Quantitative analysis of the toxicity of human amniotic fluid to cultured rat spinal cord. Pediatr Neurosurg. 1997;27:190-193.

[60] Harris MJ, Juriloff DM. An update to the list of mouse mutants with neural tube closure defects and advances toward a complete genetic perspective of neural tube closure. Birth Defects Res A Clin Mol Teratol. 2010;88:653-669.

[61] Copp AJ, Greene NDE. Genetics and development of neural tube defects. J Pathol. 2010;220:217-230.

[62] Juriloff DM, Harris MJ. A consideration of the evidence that genetic defects in planar cell polarity contribute to the etiology of human neural tube defects. Birth Defects Res A Clin Mol Teratol. 2012;94(10): 824-840.

[63] Murdoch JN, et al. Interactions between planar cell polarity genes cause diverse neural tube defects. Dis Model Mech. 2014;7:1153-1163.

[64] Amorim MR et al. Non-Latin European descent could be a requirement for association of NTDs and MTHFR variant 677C > T: a metaanalysis. Am J Med Genet. 2007;143:1726-1732.

[65] Pickell L et al. Methylenetetrahydrofolate reductase deficiency and low dietary folate increase embryonic delay and placental abnormalities in mice. Birth Defects Res A Clin Mol Teratol. 2009;85:531-541.

[66] Narisawa A, et al. Mutations in genes encoding the glycine cleavage system predispose to neural tube defects in mice and humans. Hum Mol Genet. 2012;21:1496-1503.

[67] Pai YJ, et al. Glycine decarboxylase deficiency causes neural tube defects and features of nonketotic hyperglycinemia in mice. Nat Commun. 2015;6:6388.

[68] Wald NJ et al. Blood folic acid and vitamin B12 in relation to neural tube defects. Br J Obstet Gynaecol. 1996;103(4):319-324.

[69] Imbard A et al. Neural tube defects, folic acid and methylation. Int J Environ Res Public Health. 2013;10(9):4352-4389.

[70] Denny KJ et al. Neural tube defects, folate, and immune modulation. Birth Defects Res. Part A Clin. Mol. Teratol. 2013;97(9):602-609.

[71] Bachman H et al. Holoprosencephaly and polydactyly: a possible expression of the hydrolethalus syndrome. J. Med. Genet. 1990;27(1): 50-52.

[72] Yang Y et al. Association between MTHFR C677T polymorphism and neural tube defect risks: A comprehensive evaluation in three groups of NTD patients, mothers, and fathers. Birth Defects Res. Part A Clin. Mol. Teratol. 2015; 103(6):488-500.

[73] Sharfstein JM. Folic acid antagonists during pregnancy and risk of birth defects. N. Engl. J. Med. 2001;344(12):933; author reply 934-5.

[74] Wang X et al. Role of methotrexate exposure in apoptosis and proliferation during early neurulation. J Appl Toxicol. 2014;34(8):862-869.

[75] Robert E, Guidbaud P. Maternal valproic acid and congenital neural tube defects. Lancet. 1982;320:937.

[76] Phiel CJ et al. Histone deacetylase is a direct target of valproic acid, a potent anticonvulsant, mood stabilizer, and teratogen. J Biol Chem. 2001;276: 36734-36741.

[77] Phelan SA et al. Neural tube defects in embryos of diabetic mice: role of the Pax-3 gene and apoptosis. Diabetes. 1997;46:1189-1197.

[78] Ybot-Gonzalez P et al. Convergent extension, planar cell polarity signaling and initiation of mouse neural tube closure. Development. 2007;134:789-799.

[79] Ybot-Gonzalez P et al. Neural plate morphogenesis during mouse neurulation is regulated by antagonism of BMP signaling. Development. 2007;134:3203-3211.

[80] Van Straaten HWM, Copp AJ. Curly tail: a 50-year history of the mouse spina bifida model. Anat Embryol. 2001;203: 225-237.

[81] Schoenwolf GC. Histological and ultrastructural studies of secondary neurulation of mouse embryos. Am J Anat. 1984;169:361-374.

[82] Wilson V et al. Stem cells, signals and vertebrate body axis extension. Development. 2009;136:1591-1604.

[83] Finn MA, Walker ML. Spinal lipomas: clinical spectrum, embryology, and treatment. Neurosurg Focus. 2007;23:10.

[84] Barkovich AJ, Raybaud C. Pediatric Neuroimaging. Lippincott Williams & Wilkins; 2011.

[85] McLone DG, Knepper PA. The cause of Chiari II malformation: a unified theory. Pediatr Neurosci. 1989;15:1-12.

[86] Juranek J et al. The cerebellum in children with spina bifida and Chiari II malformation: quantitative volumetrics by region. Cerebellum. 2010;9:240-248.

[87] Ware AL et al. Anatomical and diffusion MRI of deep gray matter in pediatric spina bifida. Neuroimage Clin. 2014;5:120-127.

[88] Treble-Barna A et al. Prospective and episodic memory in relation to hippocampal volume in adults with spina bifida myelo-meningocele. Neuropsychology. 2014;29:92-101.

[89] Barkovich AJ, Norman D. Anomalies of the corpus callosum: correlation with further anomalies of the brain. Am J Roentgenol. 1988;151:171-179.

[90] Crawley JT et al. Structure, integrity, and function of the hypoplastic corpus callosum in spina bifida myelomeningocele. Brain Connect. 2014;4:608-618.

[91] Herweh C et al. DTI of commissural fibers in patients with Chiari II-malformation. Neuroimage. 2009;44:306-311.

[92] Erol FS et al. How innocent is corpus callosum dysgenesis? Pediatr Neurosurg. 2013;49:24-28.

[93] Juranek J et al. Neocortical reorganization in spina bifida. Neuroimage. 2008;40:1516-1522.

[94] Del Bigio MR. Neuropathology and structural changes in hydrocephalus. Dev Disabil Res Rev. 2010;16:16-22.

[95] Hasan KM et al. White matter microstructural abnormalities in children with spina bifida myelomeningocele and hydrocephalus: a diffusion tensor tractography study of the association pathways. J Magn Reson Imaging. 2008;27:700-709.

[96] Hampton LE et al. Hydrocephalus status in spina bifida: an evaluation of variations in neuropsychological outcomes. J Neurosurg Pediatr. 2011;8:289-298.

[97] Dennis M et al. Cerebellar motor function in spina bifida meningo-myelocele. Cerebellum. 2010;9:484-498.

[98] Treble A et al. Functional significance of atypical cortical organization in spina bifida myelomeningocele: relations of cortical thickness and gyrification with IQ and fine motor dexterity. Cereb Cortex. 2013;23:2357-2369.

[99] Treble-Barna A et al. Covert orienting in three etiologies of congenital hydrocephalus: the effect of midbrain and posterior fossa dysmorphology. J Int Neuropsychol Soc. 2014;20:268-277.

[100] Taylor HB et al. Motor contingency learning and infants with spina bifida. J Int Neuropsychol Soc. 2013;19:206-215.

[101] Stubberud J et al. Emotional health and coping in spina bifida after goal management training: a randomized controlled trial. Rehabil Psychol. 2014;60:1-16.

Chapter 2

Management of Pediatric Patients with Spina Bifida

Romana Richterová, Branislav Kolarovszki and René Opšenák

Abstract

Spina bifida is a neurodevelopmental disorder and belong to most common congenital malformations. It is a neural tube defect that originates within first 28 days after conception. Although survival rate of these patients had changed rapidly within last decades, neural tube defects are still cause of substantial part of children morbidity. Occult type of spina bifida is a simple nonunion of vertebral arch without causing any symptoms. Open defects according to degree of involvement of neural tissue cause symptoms such as paralysis of lower extremities, bladder and bowel morbidity, delay in development of cognitive functions of various severity and other possible complications affecting morbidity of these patients. Early diagnosis and treatment of open spina bifida and accompaying complications is crucial and largely affects the outome. Succesfull treatment requires lifelong cooperation of a whole range of specialists and guiding of treatment by primary care doctor. Survival and quality of life are associated with acces to proper medical and surgical treatment as well as community support systems. This chapter offers overview of this topic with emphasis on general management of patients suffering from this congenital malformation.

Keywords: spina bifida, spinal dysraphism, management, spina bifida occulta, myelomeningocele, meningocele

1. Introduction

Developmental defects belong worldwide to leading causes of infant morbidity. Special interest deserve neural tube defects, that comprise anencephaly, spina bifida and encefalocele.

Spinal dysraphisms comprise a broad spectrum of congenital disorders resulting from impaired structural development of the craniospinal axis during brain and spinal cord growth and differentiation within 2nd and 6th week of gestation and proceed through a complex multistep process [1].

Spina bifida is a group of developmental disorders of neural tube. Neural tube in developing embryo forms future brain, spinal cord and their supporting structures. Under normal circumstances neural tube closes on 28th day after conception. In children with spina bifida neural tube does not develop or close properly causing dorsal defect of spine or spinal cord itself. Severity of symptoms and possible complications depends on location, size and type of defect.

Spina bifida is a complex disorder that requires multidisciplinary aproach in diagnostics, treatment and complications solving.

2. Types of spina bifida

Spina bifida or spinal dysraphism is a wide spectrum of clinical and imaging findings concerning incomplete fusion of the midline neural and bony structures during early embryogenesis. Spina bifida can be devided into closed and open forms (**Table 1**).

Closed spinal dysraphism (spina bifida occulta or ocult spinal dysraphism) is the most common type. This group of dysraphisms refers to broad spectrum of skin-covered congenital defects caused by non-union or failure to fuse of the neural tube. Clinical manifestation can range from asymptomatic simple non-union of vertebral arch taht is usually diagnosed as an incidental finding on imaging and causes no symptoms to more severe forms with progressive neurological deterioration. Closed spinal dysraphism can bez present with or without subcutaneous mass.

To closed spina bifida without subcutaneous mass belong: tethered spinal cord, dermal sinus, diastematomyelia and spinal lipoma. Closed spinal dysraphism with subcutaneous mass are: lipomyelomeningocele, lipomyelocele, terminal myelocystocele, meningocele, non-terminal myelocystocele.

Tethered spinal cord characterized by abnormal attachment of spinal cord to surrounding structures causes traction of spinal cord during growth and its ischaemisation leading to progressive motor deficit, urological and ortopedical complications [2].

Dermal sinus is a median or paramedian epithelial duct causing persistent communication connecting spinal cord with skin. It is a consequence of incomplete separation of the ectoderm from the neural crest. It is usually visible during aspection as a small pit in lumbosacral area often connected with hpertrichosis or hyperpigmentation. The duct can terminate in the soft tissue overlying spinal canal, in epidural space and, in most of the cases, directly on conus medullaris, cauda equina or fillum terminale. Newborn can display neurological deficit or can

Closed spinal dysraphism (CSD)
CSD with subcutaneous mass
Tethered cord syndrome
Dermal sinus
Diastematomyelia
Spinal lipoma
CSD without subcutaneous mass
Lipomyelomeningocele
Lipomyelocele
Terminal myelocystocele
Meningocele
Nonterminal myelocystocele
Open spinal dysraphism (OSD)
Myelomeningocele
Myelocele
Hemimyelomeningicele
Hemimyelocele

Table 1.
Types of spinal dysraphisms [3].

develop neuroinfection. Because of direct communication between skin surface and spinal canal germ can easily spread and cause meningitis or intraspinal abscess. Ultrasonography is a useful accessible first-line imaging that can show the length of the sinus. Subsequently, MR imaging is necessary. In differential diagnosis is necessary to diffentiate from sacro-coccygeal sinus that is located lower in sacral or coccygeal region and usually terminates in fascia and does not extend into sub-arachnoid space [3].

Diastematomyelia is also known as split cord malformation and it is a longitudinal split. It is mostly located between L1 and L3, less frequently between Th7 and Th12. This defect is devided according to a presence of dividing septum and single and double dural sac into two types:

Type I has common midline septum or spur, double dural sac and is symptomatic. Type II has both hemicords in a single dural sac [3].

Spinal lipoma is caused by premature separation of the ectoderm from the neural crest causing mesenchymal cells to get stick within the spinal canal. Lipoma can be extradural or intradural or their combination. Lipoma is made of adipous tissue but also contain menigeal and neural cells [4]. These lesions can expand later during life because adipocytes can increase in size easily.

Spinal lipoma can be present in 3 forms:

Filum terminale fibrolipoma – filum terminale above 2 mm thick, hyperechoic on ultrasonography, often connected with tethered cord syndrome [3].

Intradural lipoma – usually lying along midline with completely formed and propriately closed dural sac. In lumbosacral region causes often tethered cord syndrome and in cervical and thoracic regions lipoma usually causes compresion of spinal cord with subsequent symptoms [5].

Lipomyelomeningocele and **lipomyelocele** belong to closed spinal dysraphisms that present as fat-containing subcutaneous mass beginning above gluteal cleft and extending caudally in asymmetrical position [3].

Myelocystocele is a closed spinal dysraphism with dilatation of central canal of spinal cord that protrudes dorsally into the subcutaneous tissue. Spinal cord terminates in a cyst [3].

Meningocele is protrusion of meninges through a defect in vertebral column. There is a visible sac fiiled with fluid on the back but without involvement of spinal cord. There is usually minimal or none neurological impairment.

Open spinal dysraphisms are developmental anomalies that are not covered by skin and are caused by unclosure of the neural tube during primary neurulation. They are mostly diagnosed during antenatal screening by ultrasonography and are also visible during newborn physical examination. To open spinal dysraphisms belong: myelocele, myelomeningocele, hemimyelomeningocele and hemimyelocele.

Myelomeningocele is the most common and most severe type of spina bifida occuring mostly in middle or lower back (but also more cranially) forming a sac on infant's back that contains open dural layer and improperly formed spinal cord or nerve radixes. Nerve structures are extruded into the fluid-filled sac – this is called spina bifida cystica. Vertebral arches are dorsaly incomplete.

3. Epidemiology

Incidence of spina bifida varies worldwide between 1 to 10 per 1000 births [6] and between 0,17 to 6,4 per 1000 live births for myelomeningocele [7] but has differences in geogrefical regions with higher rates in less developed countries. In Europe it is around 4500 pregnancies a year that are affected by neural tube defect. Over 90% of more serious spina bifida cases is diagnosed before 22nd gestational week [8]. Overall prevalence of spina bifida is lower in countries with mandatory folic acid fortification of grain products opposite to countries with voluntary or no fortification [9, 10]. More affected are females and whites and Hispanics.

4. Etiology and pathophysiology

Detailed etiology of spina bifida is not known but it is assumed to result from a combination of more factors - genetic, nutritional and environmental risk factors. Genetic risk factor is a family history of neural tube defect. Most important nutritional factor is folate deficiency. Even though exact mechanisms leading to spina bifida are not clearly known, there are some of researchers interest [11].

4.1 Folate deficiency

Folate is a natural form of vitamin B9. Its synthetic form is folic acid. Folate is important for proper intrauterine development of fetus. Its deficiency is connested not only with spina bifida, but also with occurence of all neural tube defects. Spina bifida is significantly more common in countries without legislation regulating full-coverage folic acid fortification of the food supply and less common in world regions with mandatory folic acid fortification [9].

4.2 Positive family history of spina bifida

Genetic factors seem to play important role in etiology of spina bifida. Couples with child born with spina bifida are at higher risk of having another child born with this defect. At higher risk of having child affected by spina bifida are also women who were born with neural tube defect and also higher frequency is in twins than in singletons. All this indicates a genetic contribution to etiology. But low frequency of families with multiple neural tube defects makes research more difficult [11].

4.3 Medications

Some drugs are under suspicion in contributing to higher risk of developmental disorders of neural tube. Mostly anti-convulsants (anti-seisure mediacation), such as valproic acid, when taken during pregnancy. They probably interfere with metabolism and utilization of folate and folic acid.

4.4 Decompensated diabetes mellitus

Women with decompensated or inadequatelly compensated glucose levels during early stages of pregnancy are at higher risk of having child with spina bifida.

4.5 Obesity

Spina bifida and all neural tube defects are more common in women with obesity. It is important to have adequate body mass index also prior to pregnancy.

4.6 Hyperthermia

Increased body temperature in early stages of pregnancy due to infection or using of sauna is believed to be potencially risky for having a child with neural tube defect.

Women with present risk factors should be medicated with higher dose of folic acid preconceptionally and also during pregnancy. In women who use more risky medication (f.e. anti-seizure medication) should be pregnancy planed with switch of medication to more safe one.

5. Symptomatology

Severity of symptoms depends on type of spina bifida ranging from no symptoms in spina bifida occulta to most severe in myelomenigocele. There are also interindividual differences. Spina bifida occulta is neurologically asymptomatic because there is no involvement of neurologickal structures.

5.1 Skin lesions or visible sac

Cutaneous lesions mostly in lumbar region could be associated with spina bifida or tethered spinal cord. Visible change of skin above the defect is usually an abnormal tuft of hair, dimple, subcutaneous lipoma or a birthmark [12]. Such skin lesion could also be a symptom of spinal cord abnormality that is covered by skin.

Sacral dimple is a common skin lesion and is found in 1,8 to 7,2% of newborns [13]. However, in most of newborns it is only a simple skin lesion without any effect on neurological functions. Possitive ultrasonography findings are usually filar cyst (24,8%), echogenic filum terminale (13,5%) and low-lying spinal cord (11,7%). Some literary sources consider filar cyst as a normal finding [14].

Simple solitaire sacral dimple in asymptomatic newborn with diameter less than 5 mm located no more than 25 mm above anal opening have extremely low risk of having spinal abnormality [15]. Considering this very low risk (approx. 0,34%), more recent guidelines state that sipmple solitaire non risky sacral dimples do not require additional imaging – only in case they are atypical, associated with other skin lesions or multiple. On the other hand around 86% of spinal dysraphisms are associated with overlying cutaneous lesion [16].

Open defect is mostly situated in the lumbar region and is characterized by opened spinal canal along more vertebras. At birth meninges, spinal nerves and spinal cord protrude above surrounding skin level forming a sac. This sac could be also covered by skin. These open defects are easily recognized whereas smaller or closed defects can present only by overlying cutaneous lesions [17].

5.2 Paraparesis

Degree of neurological impairment, walking disability and muscle weaknes depends on severity and extent of the defect, as well as on accuracy of prenatal or postnatal treatment. Neurological deficit varies from mild paraparesis to paraplegia. Myelomeningocele is the most common congenital anomaly causing physical disability [18].

According to level of defect there are various degrees of motor disability (**Table 2**). Patients with thoracic defect have flacid lower extremities, patients with high-lumbar defect usually can perform flexion in hip joint, in middle-lumbar defect also extension in knee, in low-lumbar defect is also foot dorsiflection present and sacral defect usually allows to perform also plantar flexion of foot [20].

Neurological deficit in patients with spina bifida is thought to be result of the primary insult - the congenital anomaly and the second - from direct exposure of spinal cord to amniotic fluid and intrauterine trauma [21].

Level of lesion	Muscle function	Ambulation
Thoracic High Lumbar	Lack quadriceps function	Children – ambulation with hip spanning orthosis (hip-knee- ankle – foot orthosis or reciprocating gait orthosis) Adults – majority require wheelchair
Low lumbar	Lack function of gluteus maximus and medius Retain quadriceps and medial hamstring function	Require crutches for ambulation Most retain comunity ambulation as adults
Sacral	Retain quadriceps and gluteus medius function	
High sacral	Lack gastrocnemius function	Ambulate with ankle-foot orthosis and no support
Low sacral	Retain gastrocnemius function	Ambulate without braces or support

Table 2.
Functional outcome according to level of spinal dysraphism [19].

In a study with 50 years follow up of walking ability half of the patients with severe spina bifida was able to walk for 50 m butthis ability declined with age to 27% in the age of 50 years [22].

5.3 Urinary dysfunction

Nerve damage in neural tube defect leads to loss of sensation and bladder sphincter control. Very common is neurogenic bladder that leads to symptoms such as urinary retencion, overflow incontinence, urgency, frequency and nocturia. Possible complications are incontinence, repeated or chronic urinary infections, hydronephrosis and in later stages renal damage [23] that all leads to diminished quality of life [24].

5.4 Bowel dysfunction

Most of patients living with the diagnosis of spina bifida have some degree of bowel problems called neurogenic bowel dysfuntion. The lack of bowel movement results in obstipation and lack of anal sphincter control leads to intermitent or continual incontinence [23]. Bowel dysfunction leads to decreased life quality [19, 25].

6. Complications

Possible complication affect in some degree most of patients with open forms of spina bifida. The severity of complications depend on extent of defect and also on timing of treatment. Fetal surgery gives better prognosis.

6.1 Hydrocephalus

The majority of infants with open neural tube defects also has hydrocephalus [26]. Hydrocephalus is defined as an active distension of the ventricular system resulting from inadequate passage of cerebrospinal fluid at some point from its production within ventricles to its absorption into the systemic circulation [27]. In infants it is a condition with ventricular enlargement that leads to rapid growth of head circumference and requires surgical intervention [28]. According to observations only 1 out of 6 infants with myelomenongocele has symptoms of raised intracranial pressure at birth and 1 out of 8 has head circumference above 98th percentille at birth [29]. Many infants develop ventriculomegally that leads to increase of head circumference after postnatal closure of open spina bifida. Slight ventricular enlargement with stable neurological status could be indication for conservative observation – radiological and clinical. Rapidly developed ventricullomegaly with worsening of neurological status and signs of intracranial hypertension requires quick neurosurgical intervention [26].

Surgical treatment possibilities are insertion of ventriculo-peritoneal shunt and endoscopic third ventriculostomy with cauterisation of choroid plexus. Minority of cases is indicated for conservative treatment – only those with relatively stable ventriculomegally [26]. Infants who underwent fetal surgical repair of myelomeningocele were less likely to require ventriculo-peritoneal shunting [30].

6.2 Complications of ventriculo-peritoneal drainage

Presence of hydrocephalus in children with open spina bifida requires placement of ventriculo-peritoneal shunt in most of the cases. Proper function of shunt is inevitable. Unfortunately, shunt related complications are frequent – mainly shunt malfunction and infection. About 95% of patients who required shunt placement have to undergo at least one shunt revision [26]. Symptoms of shunt-related complications are: headache, irritability, confusion, somnolency, nausea, vomiting, feeding problems, fixed downward gaze, seizures. In case of shunt infections also symptoms like higher body temperature, redness along the shunt catheters, elevated blood parameters of infections.

6.3 Chiari malformation type II

Myelomeningocele as the most severe open defect is almost invariably associated with this malformation. Chiari malformation type II is a group of disorders that includes herniation of fetal developing cerebellum upwards into the middle cranial fossa or downwards into cervical spinal canal. This malformation is often associated with other abnormalities such as: brainstem kinking, abnormal forth ventricle location and syringomyelia [30]. The research on animal models shows that chronic intrauterine leakage of cerebrospinal fluid can lead to Chiari II malformation [31]. It is common brain malformation in children with myelomeningocele. This malformation worsens the cerebrospinal fluid circulation leading to progression of hydrocephalus. Chiari malformation type II can present with rapidly present symptoms such as: breathing problems or apnoea, bradycardia, swallowing problems and other cranial nerves dysfunction when descending cerebellum presses on brainstem [26]. Under rare circumstances can lead to indication of decompression of craniocervical junction. Chiari malformation type II, its presence and severity can in huge extent determine the outcome of patients [26]. Chiari II malformation is significantly less severe in infants who underwent fetal surgery for myelomeningocele [30]. Improvement of this malformation and subsequent decrease in hydrocephalus in children with prenatal repair of myelomeningocele support the theory of relationship between continual intrauterine abnormal leakage of cerebrospinal fluid and subsequent development of Chiari II malformation and hydrocephalus and underline the importance of fetal surgery [26, 30].

6.4 Tethered spinal cord

Tethered spinal cord is a neurological disorder that is caused by abnormal attachment of the spinal cord to surrounding structures. In case of patients with myelomeningocele spinal cord is mostly attached to scar from previous operation [32]. Symptoms are caused by increased tension and stretch-induces dysfunction of the caudal spinal cord and conus and include motor and sensitive dysfunction, gait abnormalities, symptoms of cauda equina syndrome and urological symptoms [12, 32].

Filum terminale lipoma can cause cord tethering, lipoma is the most common cause of thick filum terminale. That is why detection of abnormal thickening of filum terminale is important. Initial detection is usually performed by ultrasonography [2] followed by MR imaging [12]. Tethered cord syndrome must be suspected when conus medullaris is placed dorsaly in the spinal canal and terminates below the superior aspect of L3 vertebral body. Also thickened filum terminale can be present. MR imaging is indicated in ultrasonography evidence of tethered cord or in case of doubts [3].

Although some patients with anatomic cord tethering do not develop symptoms, most of the patients are symptomatic and do not naturally improve without surgical untethering. Neurosurgical intervention is the treatment of choice, though with varying results [33]. Timing of the surgery is also important – early intervention after symptom development is necessary for recovery or at least improval of neurological functions. Early surgical intervention as a prevention of further neurological damage requires early diagnostics [12].

6.5 Meningitis

Infants with open neural tube defects can experience meningitis – inflammation of brain and spinal cord surrounding meninges. Meningitis could develop as a consequence of open defect, as a complication of surgical procedures as well as a complication of shunting procedures. In case of bacterial meningitis there is a need for massive antibiotic therapy.

6.6 Urological complications

Most of the patients with severe spinal dysraphism suffer from neuropathic bladder impairment [24]. As the nerve damage causes urological complication by means of neurgenic bladder, this situation also brings specific possible complications. Usual problem is urinary retention that could lead to overflow incontinence, renal damage and urinary tract infections, that could be repeated or chronic and often requires antibiotic treatment.

It is necessary to maintain proper urine derivation with no residual urine left. These patients require long time follow up by urologist. Urological complications and renal disease as a consequence is very common cause of higher morbidity mainly in older children and adults with open spinal defect. Severe bladder mortality is most frequently present in patients with huge spinal defects without covering membrane. This verifies the theory of increased damage of nerve roots from direct exposure to amniotic fluid [34].

6.7 Gastrointestinal complications

One of the most common problems of patient with spina bifida in adulthood is neuropathic bowel dysfunction with constipation and incontinence, but these patients also often suffer from dysphagia – mainly patients with brain stem compression.

Brain and spinal cord nerves modulate activity of enteric nervous system. Patients with severe and highly located forms of open spina bifida and resulting Chiari II malformation have impaired function of nerves leading to dysfunction of gastrointestinal tract mobility. Gastrointestinal problem that these patients suffer from is diminished bowel movements causing obstipation or opposite also diarrhea. Patients often suffer from anal incontinence from mild to severe degree [19].

Patients with large and high located myelomeningocele often suffer from dysphagia. Development of dysphagia in children with myelomeningocele is caused by cervicomedulary kinking and brainstem compression due to crowding in the posterior fossa in Chiari II malformation. Dysphagia leads to swallowing difficulties, feeding difficulties, failure to thrive, bronchopulmonary complications and later to peptic ulcer disease [34, 35].

6.8 Bronchopulmonal complications

Children with large and high located myelomeningocele display also other complications such as Chiari II malformation that often leads to dysfagia. Severe dysphagia causes swallowing and feeding problems that might cause complications as aspiration pneumonia, pulmonary disease, reactive airway disease, bronchiectasis, stridor or apnoea [35]. Although almost all children with open spina bifida live into adulthood, patient suffering with brainstem dysfunction leading to such bronchopulmonary complications are at higher risk of fatal complications [34].

Children with thoracic and thoracolumbar levels of defect might in some cases also have impaired function of the accessory respiratory muscles. They also often have scoliosis that could lead to reduced forced vital capacity of the lungs [36].

6.9 Orthopedic complications

Orthopedics deal in patients with spina bifida with congenital and acquired deformities. Because of weak muscles of spine and lower extremities, these patients with open spinal defects can present with variety of orthopedic problems. Most frequently occuring problems are: scoliosis, kyphosis, muscle contractions, bone and joints deformities, hip dislocation, abnormal growth and talipes (club foot) [37].

Scoliosis is present in almost all children with severe and highly located myelomeningocele. Children born without covering membrane of the defect tend to have neuromuscular imbalance and spinal cord tethering which are conditions leading to scoliosis. Severe paraparesis leading to full-time use of wheelchair also enables occurrence of scoliosis [34]. Scoliosis also leads to pelvic obliquity with subsequent changes in sitting balance and contributes to unequal pressure during sitting. This factor together with lack of sensitivity leads to skin breakdowns [36]. One of the most important factors for maintaining ambulation in adulthood is strength of quadriceps and hamstring muscles [11].

6.10 Latex allergy

Many patients with open spinal defects are at higher risk of latex allergy. This means allergic reaction to natural rubber and latex products. Symptoms could be mild – such as rush, sneezing, itching, conjunctivitis and rhinitis, as well as very severe condition – anaphylaxis, that is potentially life threatening situation. This is a potential reason for using latex-free gloves at labor and also at giving care to these patients. Latex allergy could also lead to perioperative complications [11].

6.11 Sleep disorders

Children and adults with open neural tube defects often suffer from sleep disorders, from which sleep apnoea is the most severe one potentially affecting life quality. These patients should undergo evaluation of sleep disorders.

6.12 Wound heeling

Because of lack of skin sensitivity below the level of open spinal defect, patients do not properly feel small wounds or sores on their lower extremities, buttocks and back region. That is reason that these small wounds may develop into more severe wounds that are more difficult to heal and may sometimes cause generalized infection. Skin breakdowns are also consequence of friction and pressure related to the use of orthotic aids that assist in positioning and ambulation as well as constant pressure on insensitive skin due to immobility, especially with increasing body size and weight [38].

Many patients with open spinal defect have altered sitting balance due to paralysis of abdominal, thoracic and lumbar extensor musculature. Due to this imbalance together with insensate skin leads to frequent skin breakdowns [36].

6.13 Neurocognitive disorders and educational status

Many children with severe forms of spina bifida suffer from specific learning disabilities, such as dyslexia, dyscalculia, problems with paying attention. Patients with less severe forms of spinal dysraphism and with lower levels of defect have higher chance to obtain higher education and better employment and insurance status [19].

6.14 Psychological problems

Patients with open spinal defect prone more to develop depression or suffer from anxiety. Attaining early ambulation provides psychological benefits even if the child later becomes sitter [11].

7. Diagnostics

Early diagnosis of spina bifida is crucial. This applies to open forms. It is known that closed spinal defect that affects only vertebral arch is often just incidental finding without clinical correlate. Early diagnose of open spinal defect gives better chances for better prognosis and for fetal surgery. In some sever cases it could lead to decision of termination of pregnancy.

7.1 Prenatal diagnostics

Screening of neural tube defect is part of routine prenatal screening. Each pregnant women is offered to undergo screening tests. Widely used screening tests during pregnancy are blood tests fetal ultrasonography. In special cases can also amniocentesis be indicated. Fetal MR imaging is used to verified neural tube defect in cases when fetal surgery is planned.

7.1.1 Blood tests

Initial wide screening for neural tube defects is made by blood tests. It is important to know that this test can have false positive as well as false negative results.

7.1.2 Maternal serum alpha-fetoprotein (MSAFP) test

A sample of maternal blood is taken for this test. Test determines the level of alpha-fetoprotein (AFP) in maternal serum. This protein is produced by fetal tissues and in normal production only small levels of this protein reaches mother's bloodstream. In abnormally high production of AFP, higher level of MSAFP can be detected.

Normal MSAFP level does not absolutely exclude diagnosis of spina bifida. On the other hand high MSAFP levels could be caused by miscalculation of fetal age or multifetus gravidity. In case of positive MSAFP test it is usually repeated. If the level remains high there is an indication for further evaluation, usually by ultrasonography. AFP test can be a part of triple screen test that is used for screening of neural tube defects but also other organs abnormalities.

7.1.3 Fetal ultrasonography

This diagnostic tool is widely and successfully used screening imaging tool. It is also accurate tool for early diagnostics of open spina bifida. Morphological ultrasound is made three time during pregnancy in each trimester. The first two ultrasounds are most important for early diagnostics. First examination by ultrasonography is performed usually between 11th to 14th gestational week. Second trimester examination is usual between 18th to 22nd week and this imaging is most important for assessment of correct fetal morphology and evaluation of signs of present spina bifida or hydrocephalus [2]. More advanced ultrasonograph could detect also milder forms of spina bifida and in experienced hands could be also useful in evaluation of severity of defect. Children with higher spinal lesions on prenatal ultrasound have more serious motor impairment [20].

7.1.4 Amniocentesis

Amnicentesis could be indicated after positive ultrasonography. This test is performed by needle inserted transabdominally under ultrasound control to amniotic cavity to take a sample from amniotic fluid. Amniotic fluid can be tested for AFP levels. Cells from amniotic fluid are used for genetic examination to rule out genetic abnormalities causing spina bifida, although genetically associated spina bifida is rare. This needs to be taken into account in decision making as the procedure of amniocentesis caries also risks.

7.1.5 Fetal MRI

Fetal MR imaging is a powerful diagnostic tool for evaluation of neuroaxis. It plays an important role in prenatal diagnosis, treatment planning and follow up [39]. Fetal MRI is used for determining the level of spinal defect and for selection of candidates for fetal surgery [34]. Fetal MRI is used in cases where prenatal screening and ultrasonography is positive. Open spinal defect in higher levels of spine is more often connected with increased fetal ventricular size [40]. Morphological evaluation by fetal MR imaging provides valuable information for prognosis and possible complications. Higher defects are frequently associated with dysfagia and absence of membrane covering defect is commonly associated with scoliosis and high risk of severe bladder dysfunction. Location and size of defect correlates with severity of motor deficiency, patients with higher and larger defects are predicated for full-time wheelchair use. Lenght and width of defect of the body defect are measured as segment span and interpediculate distance [34].

7.2 Postnatal diagnostics

Ultrasonography is a safe and effective screening method that is commonly used in screening system of the newborns. It is noninvasive imaging method that does not require sedation of newborn without exposure to radiation [12]. Newborns with physiological finding on ultrasonography do not require any further imaging evaluation. On the other hand, positive finding on ultrasonography require more detailed imaging performed by MR imaging [41].

7.2.1 Ultrasonography

Ultrasonography is the first-line survey for the assessment of spinal cord abnormalities. During the first six months of life non-ossificated vertebral arches and cartilagineous posterior elements provide acoustic window for detained imaging of spinal canal with its content and surrounding soft tissues [17].

Ultrasonography of the spinal cord in infants is very effective tool for imaging of spine and spinal cord compared to postossification [3, 12]. Major indication of spinal ultrasonography in selected group of newborns is possible detection of tethered cord syndrome. Progress of ossification in time makes ultrasonography more difficult [12].

Indications for spinal ultrasonography in newborns are: cutaneous lesions on the back (such as hypertrichosis, subcuteaneous lipoma, sacral sinus, sacral dimple), spinal deformity, neurological abnormality (paraparesis, neurogenic bladder or bowel dysfunction), spinal trauma during delivery and syndromes with associated compression of spinal cord [41].

Spinal ultrasonography is performed in infant in lying prone position with the upper body higher than lower and in flexed spine (curved over pillow). This position offers better acoustic window. Imaging is performed with linear transducer through longitudinal and axial plane scans from craniocervical junction to coccyx [3].

The main structures that must be identified are: conus medularis, filum terminale, cauda equina and spinal roots, central echo complex and subarachnoid spaces. Tip of conus medularis is in newborns usually located L1 and L2 interspace, occasionally on the level of superior end plate of L3. Filum terminale is a band of fibrous tissue that extends from the conus to the caudal end of spinal canal. At the level of L5 and S1 it should be less than 2 mm thick and should be predominantly hypoechoic with a bright hyperechoic periphery. Cauda equina and spinal roots must move according to the pulsatile production of cerebrospinal fluid, as the ultrasonography provides live image of the structures. Central echo-complex is train-line hyperechogenicity provided by the interface of the two margins of spinal canal. It needs to be detectable at all levels of spine and the space must be regular along entire extension. The subarachnoid space is anechoic and does not contain structures except spinal cord and nerve roots [3].

In order to avoid unnecessary further imagings it is important to know some anatomical variations that are considered physiological. Some of them are: mild thickening of the epidural fat, mild thickening of the filum terminale (between 1 and 2 mm), malformation of the coccyx with palpable prominence in the sacral region, transient dilatation of the central canal (usually disappears during the first weeks).

7.2.1.1 Persistence of ventriculus terminalis

Also known as fifth ventricle. It refers to mild cystic dilatation of the terminal part of spinal cord canal due to incomplete regression of embryonic ventriculus terminalis in the conus medularis. This condition is usually asymptomatic, but in some patients could cause low back pain, sciatica or urinary bladder dysfunction [3].

7.2.2 Other imaging methods

As ultrasonography of the brain and spine is quick and good available it is the bet diagnostic first-line tool. But for proper imaging of brain, spine and supporting structures for evaluation of extent of the defect, treatment planning and estimation of prognosis there is a need for use of other diagnostic methods. After detailed ultrasonography newborns with more severe spinal defects undergo MR imaging of spine. In open spinal defects with a risk of hydrocephalus newborns undergo CT or MR imaging of the brain according to clinical need with a detection of serious neuroimaging findings, such as ventriculomegally, tonsilar descent, hind brain abnormalities, nodular heterotopia of gray matter and corpus callosum abnormalities – such as aplasia, hypoplasia/partial aplasia with or without dysplasia [23].

8. Termination of pregnancy

Termination of pregnancy with severe fetal anomalies is a controversal issue with many moral and ethical controversies. Indication for termination of such pregnancy is a medical decision but as well moral choice of mother or parents. This moral choice is affected by religion beliefs, legislation, cultural values and socio-economical status [42]. Around 40% of mothers decide to continue with pregnancy after diagnose of severe open spinal dysraphism [23].

9. Treatment

Treatment of spina bifida depends on severity of primary defect. Occult forms of spina bifida usually do not require any treatment. All other forms are indicated for surgical repair.

There has been a significant improval of patient outcomes in the past 50 years because of multidisciplinary approach with an increased life quality of patients and prolonged life expectancy [43]. But though survival has changed significantly within past decades, there has not been significant improval of neurological outcome [44]. In struggle to ameliorate the neurological outcome fetal surgery seems to be a promise. If fetal surgery is not indicated newborn needs to be operated soon after birth.

As the spina bifida is a complex problem, also treatment needs to be complex and include also treatment of complications.

9.1 Fetal surgery

Neurological deficit in patients with spina bifida is thought to be result of two circumstances – the primary insult is the congenital anomaly and the second is from direct exposure of spinal cord to amniotic fluid and intrauterine trauma. This hypothesis is the rationale for preventing secondary damage to spinal cord by fetal surgery [21].

Fetal surgery in fetus with open type of spina bifida, though risky, is a promising procedure in improval of neurological outome. This procedure has to take place before completed 26th week of gestation. Indication for fetal surgery is a result of multidisciplinary decision. Fetal surgery should be performed only in centres experienced with fetal surgery equipped by neonatology intensive care unit. It requires cooperation of more specialists: pediatric neurosurgeon, gynecologist, fetal surgeon, fetal cardiologist and neonatologist. During this procedure uterus needs to be surgically exposed, opened and spinal cord and meninges of the fetus are closed and covered by skin. In some cases this procedure can be performed less invasively by means of fetoscope.

Prenatal surgery of fetuses with open spina bifida – myelomeningocele before 26th weeks of gestation leads to lower incidence of postnatal presence of Chiari II malformation or its lower severity and less amount of infants with myelomeningocele requiring ventriculo-peritoneal drainage for hydrocephalus. Other abnormalities accompanying Chiari II malformation – such as kinking of brainstem and dislocation of forth ventricle are less frequent in infants who underwent prenatal repair of myelomeningocele [30]. Children after fetal surgery are less likely to need mobility aids, such as crutches. But fetal surgery still remains a risky procedure with possible pregnancy complications such as preterm rupture of membranes and premature delivery before 34th week of gestation in almost half of the cases that underwent fetal surgery [30]. Persistence of Chiari II malformation with descendent herniation on MR imaging 6 weeks after prenatal repair is a predictor of need for postnatal surgical hydrocephalus treatment [45].

Since prenatal surgery might bring more favorable results but carries risk of premature birth, parents facing decision about prenatal versus postnatal repair, need to get reliable and up-to-date information to make this difficult and necessary choice [23].

9.2 Postnatal surgery

Myelomeningicele and meningicele if not treated prenataly, need to be surgically treated as soon as possible within the first days after delivery [46]. Early surgery gives better chances for good outcome. Another reason for early surgery is diminishing the risk of infection of exposed neural structures. During surgical procedure surgeon closes spinal cord a creates a meningeal layer around spinal cord and covers defect with muscular and skin layer. In case of newborn with symptoms of intracranial hypertension, ventriculoperitoneal shunt can be immediately implanted to treat hydrocephalus.

A meta-analysis of two prospective studies showed no significant difference in neurological outcome between prenatal and postnatal surgical repair, but suggested improved independent ambulation at 30 months of age in children following prenatal repair [47]. Surgical complications are cerebro-spinal fluid leakage, infection and wound healing complications [23].

9.3 Treatment of complications

As the irreparable nerve damage has already occurred during abnormal development all treatment modalities aim to minimize resulting neurological deficit and to treat complications and to exclude them form having impact on life quality and overall survival. Treatment of complications usually begins right after birth. Some patients require repeated surgeries.

Although advances in treatment of spinal defect, such as fetal surgery and active screening and early treatment of complications have rapidly changed survival of these patients, complications are main cause of mortality of myelomeningocele patients. Most severe complications with possible impact on survival are brain stem dysfunction, hydrocephalus, shunt related complications and ventriculitis in children and renal disease in later life.

9.4 Treatment of hydrocephalus

Hydrocephalus may be present at birth with symptoms of active hydrocephalus leading to raised intracranial pressure. In such conditions hydrocephalus needs to be treated immediately. In cases without acute symptomatic hydrocephalus could be initial decision of observation. In case of rising symptoms of hydrocephalus it needs to be treated. Typical procedure is insertion of ventriculoperitoneal shunt, in which cerebrospinal fluid is being drained to peritoneal cavity where it is resorbed. This shunt system consists of ventricular catheter, ventil with chamber and distal peritoneal catether. This type of drainage is most common. If there is a contraindication for drainage of cerebrospinal fluid to peritoneal cavity, it can be rarely drained to pleural cavity, right atrium of heart through venous system and very occasionally to gall bladder. Newer method is endoscopical procedure – third ventriculostomy in cases with stenosis of Sylvian aqueduct with cauterisation of choroid plexus to minimize production of cerebrospinal fluid. Possible complications of shunt systems, such as malfunction or infection usually require shunt revision. During growth children usually require revision with prolongation at least once [23].

9.5 Bladder and bowel management

Patients with open spina bifida need to be regularly evaluated for bladder and bowel functions to minimize the risk of complications and organ damage. Regular blood tests, ultrasound, kidney function tests, urodynamic assessment and X-rays need to be performed.

Urinary and bowel complications are associated with diminished life quality of patients [25]. Degree of continence and management techniques differ by type of spina bifida and age of patient.

Urological management consists of medications, proper and sufficient urine derivation – using catheters to empty urinary bladder if necessary and some surgical procedures. Patients with overactive bladder may require anticholinergic medical therapy. Antibiotic medication for treatment of urinary infection and in indicated cases also as a prophylaxis [23, 24]. Some patient also require clean intermittent catheterisation – CIC [23]. Surgical procedures used in these patients are: bladder augmentation, continent cathetrizable urinary channel, cutaneous vesicostomy, bladder outlet operation for continence and urinary stone removal. Used bladder management techniques are: indwelling catether, CIC, cutaneous vesicostomy, urostomy into external appliance, condom catheter and use of Credé maneuver. Some patients are left incontinent in diaper and some have spontaneous controlled voiding [24].

Urinary management also changes with age of these patients. Chance for spontaneous voiding decreases with age. Daily use of antibiotics as a prophylaxis is rare, but more common in adults. Almost half of patients uses antimuscarinic medication and this is more frequent in children and younger age groups. Alpha adrenergic receptor agonist and antagonist medication to improve continence and voiding is rare [24]. One fourth of adults have undergone bladder augmentation. Creation of continent cathetrizable channel (Mitrofanoff or Monti), cutaneous vesicostomy and bladder outlet operation are more common in adults compared to school children and adults. History of surgery for urinary stones is more prevalent in adult age group. Use of CIC is less frequent in school children than in older age groups and is more common in patients with severe open spinal dysraphism. Management by indwelling catheter, condom catheter, Credé maneuver or urostomy bag (incontinent diversion) is overall less frequent but from age groups is more common in adults. Patients with spina bifida are more likely to develop urinary stones and this risk increases with age, so higher rate of urinary stone removal in adults is not unexpected [24].

Bladder continence is reported to increase by age. Around one third of patients is continent in school age but almost half of the patients in adult age [24]. Though urinary incontinence affects life quality, it has lower impact than bowel incontinence [48].

Bowel management consists of oral medications, antiemetics, suppositories and sometimes also manual derivation of stools by digital stimulation and disimpaction of stools. Other management possibilities are also use of standard rectal enema, cone enema and mini enema [19]. Though rarely, some cases are treated with anal plug [23].

Dramatic improvement of life quality of patients with severe anal incontinence, severe constipation and no anal control can experience with antegrade continence enema – ACE, that is minimally invasive surgical procedure [23].

Other surgical procedures for treatment of neurogenic bowel dysfunction are: cecostomy button or tube, cecostomy button closure, colostomy and ileostomy [19].

Type of used bowel management tool may also differ by age. Use of oral medication is low or insufficient in all age groups. Timed evacuation and suppositories are more used in small children and their use decreases with age. Standard rectal enemas are more used in school children and adults and less by adolescents. Cone and mini enemas are more used in school children and less by adolescents and adults. Antegrade enemas through a surgically created chanel or a cecostomy button and tube are more used in adolescent age than in childhood and adulthood. Digital stimulation and disimpaction is used by small number of patients and mostly used in adults. Higher prevalence of colostomy is in adults. Ileostomy is less frequently performed [19]. Degree of continence and sufficiency of incontinence control has great impact on life quality of patients with spina bifida [19].

9.6 Treatment of orthopedic complications

The mail goal of orthopedic treatment in patients with spina bifida is to correct deformities that may prevent the patient from using orthoses to ambulate during childhood [11]. Orthopedic complications are common in patients with spinal defects, mostly congenital and acquired deformities. Frequent congenital defermities are kyphosis, hemivertebra, teratologic hip dislocation, clubfoot and vertical talus. Acquired developmental deformities are related to the level of defect and are caused by muscle imbalance, paralysis and lack of sensitivity in lower extremities, such as contractures, calcaneus and cavovarus. Orthopedical complications may also be a consequence of surgical intervention – for example in postoperative tethered cord syndrome [11].

Orthopedical surgical interventions are most common within first 5 years of life, especially within the first year of life – mostly due to presence of congenital deformities that require surgical correction [38].

Deformities of **hip joint** are mostly contracture, subluxation and dislocation and also rotational deformity of the lower extremity, such as internal or external torsion. This deformity is a result of muscle imbalance and paralysis of the supporting muscles. Untreated deformity could lead to pelvic obliquity and compensatory spinal deformity.

Knee joint can be affected by flexion or extension contracture, valgus deformity or late knee instability and pain. Contractures are more common in patients with higher location of spinal defect. Flexion contracture is a result of gradual contracture of the hamstrings with contracture of the posterior knee capsule due to prolonged sitting and quadriceps weakness or spasticity of the hamstrings and quadriceps weakness due to tethered spinal cord. Flexion deformity can be present in ambulatory and also non-ambulatory patients. Surgical release of the hamstrings, gastrocnemius and posterior capsule can decrease the angle of contracture and improve the ambulation.

Extension contractures are much less common and occurs secondary to unopposed quadriceps function in weak hamstrings, extensive bracing in extension or surgical treatment for flexion contracture, but most of the cases are congenital and often also with teratogenic hip dislocation or clubfoot. Initial treatment is usually serial casting attempting to achieve satisfactory knee flexion that is around 90 degree. If the contraction interferes with gait and is persistent, usually VY plasty of quadriceps is performed with good results. In non-ambulatory patients in whom the contraction causes difficulties with sitting, tenotomy of patellar tendon is an option.

Deformity of the knee joint is a result of static forces of positioning, fibrosis of the surrounding muscles, muscle imbalance around knee joint and fracture malunion. Valgus knee deformity is more common in patients with low-lumbar or sacral dysraphism and leads to instability, pain and acceleration of arthrosis in adulthood.

Torsional deformities of femur and tibia are frequent in patients with severe spinal dysraphims and presents more severe problem for ambulatory patients. Femoral torsion is present normally in all newborns initially, but in children with severe spina bifida does not decrease with growth due to abnormal gait and activity. Tibial torsion is more common. Internal torsion is congenital and frequently associated with clubfoot and external torsion is acquired secondary to muscle imbalance. Initial treatment is usually ankle-foot orthosis with twister cables. If not successful, internal torsion of tibia can be treated by rotational osteotomy and severe cases of external torsion by internal rotational osteotomy of the tibia.

Foot and ankle deformities lead to problems with effective ambulation, cause difficulties with bracing and shoe wear, affect cosmetic appearance of foot and can cause skin irritation leading to pressure sores [49]. Surgical intervention is usually tendor excision or osteotomy for bony deformity followed by use of ankle-foot orthosis during day and splint during night. Arthrodesis in these deformities should be strictly avoided because stiffness resulting from fusion in combination with insensate foot can cause neuropathic skin changes [49].

Clubfoot is the most common foot deformity in spina bifida patients [50]. Factors that contributes to development of clubfoot are spasticity, intrauterine positioning, contractures and muscle imbalance. Treatment methods that could be used are: serial manipulations and long-leg casting to gradually correct deformity and tenotomy of the Achilles tendon followed by foot abduction bracing for several years. If this treatment is ineffective there is an indication for double osteotomy – closing wedge osteotomy of the cuboid with an opening wedge osteotomy of the medial cuneiform.

Equinus is also frequent deformity. Spasticity probably plays the most important role in it etiology. In prevention regular routine of passive stretching with a night-time ankle-foot orthosis is used. Surgical treatment is indicated in patients with unbraceable foot with skin breakdowns. Mild deformities respond to Achilles tendon excision, severe contractures require radical posterior release in the posterior tibiotalar and talocalcaneal joints.

Another contracures occuring in spina bifida patients are vertical talus, calcaneus or calcaneovalgus, ankle valgus, hindfoot valgus, cavus, varus and cavovarus [49].

More severe cases may require surgical repair – correction of ankle or foot deformity, correction of congenital foot deformity, correction of equinus contracture, tendon excisions, correction of scoliosis, osteotomy for correction of bony deformity, osteotomy of femur, pelvic osteotomy, reduction of hip dislocation, release of contracture of hip or knee joint, spinal fusion and corrective osteotomies for scoliosis. Spina bifida patients are at higher risk of postoperative complications such as wound infection, delayed union or malunion, skin breakdowns and post-immobilization fractires. For post-surgical imobilisation custom-molded total body splint should be used and spica total body cast should be avoided [11].

Measures of muscle strenght are key for surgical management of orthopedic patients [38]. Better functional effect in patients with spina bifida is a result of better understanding of impact of radiologically diagnosed deformities on functional effect within last decades and their earlier treatment as a prevention of deterioration [11].

9.7 Complications of mobility

Due to present paraparesis in almost all cases, patient usually need mobility aids, such as: crutches, braces, walkers or even wheelchair at least for some time during growth. These mobility aids together with regular physiotherapy can help the child to become more independent. For daily functioning some aids could be used such as walking frames, commode chairs and bath chairs.

According to functional mobility ambulatory outcome could be:

Community ambulator who walks indoors and outdoors for most activities and may need crutches or braces.

Household ambulator who walks only indoors with help of aids and may use a wheelchair for some activities.

Therapeutic ambulator who can walk only in therapy session, sometimes with help of appartuses.

Nonambulator who exclusively uses a wheelchair for most of his activities [38].

Various factors affect ability to ambulate, most important of those are: level of neurological impairment, hip deformity, scoliosis, foot and ankle deformity, age and presence of obesity [11].

Almost all patients with severe forms of spinal dysraphism with exception of some patients with low sacral lesions will require use of orthoses in ambulation from indications, such as maintanance of alignment, prevention of deformity, correction of flexible deformity, facilitation of independent mobility and protection of insensitive limb.

In children with defect in thoracic and high-lumbar regions around age of 12 months if child controls head and neck position, usually standing frame is prescribed, later hip-knee-ankle-foot orthosis and reciprocating gait orthosis.

Patients with low-lumbar and sacral spinal dysrahpism usually require solid ankle-foot orthosis as it substitues for weak or absent ankle plantar flexors and dorsiflexors. Use of forearm crutches should be considered as well, as these patients often display weakness of hip extensors and abductors. Patients with internal or external rotational deformity can benefit from ankle-foot orthosis with twister cables. Also knee-ankle-foot orthosis can be used in patients with excessive valgus stress at the knee joint who are too young for correctional osteotomy.

9.8 Wound healing and prevention

Skin problems are very common in patients suffering from spina bifida [50]. As the skin sensitivity is affected in children and adults born with open spina bifida they are more likely to develop various skin problems. Blisters, soles, calluses and burns on lower extremities are frequent. When found late this skin problems can lead to serious problems of complicated healing.

The most common site of pressure sores are sacrum, ischial tuberosity, greater trochanter and feet. Severe complication of skin breakdown and pressure sores is osteomyelitis of the underlying bone. When wound does not heal with appropriate soft tissue care, underlying deep infection must be suspected and diagnosed by laboratory and radiograph findings. Antibiotic treatment is indicated, in more severe cases also surgical debridement. Last therapeutical opportunity in severe non-healing deep wounds causing sepsis is amputation with preservation as much lenght of the extremity as possible [49].

Parents and caregives need to prevent bed sores – avoid lying on one side too long, prevent sun burns and regularly control skin of back and lower extremities at least once a day. In case of new orthosis even more often. In older children it is necessary to control if the shoes fit properly. Barefoot walking should be avoided, especially on rough and hot surfaces. Self-adhesive foam pads can be used over pressure points [49].

Interventions of plastic surgeon within first year of life are mostly skin flaps and skin grafts associated with spinal closure. Need for surgery due to complications of wound healing is increasing with age.

In case of more severe bad healing wounds there is sometimes necessary to perform surgical debridement of skin wound, incision and drainage of abscess, skin flap operations, flap grafts, skin grafting, reduction of callus and revisions of skin scars [38].

9.9 Sexual dysfunction

Because of nerve damage patients born with open spina bifida defect suffer from sexual dysfunction in adolescence and adulthood. This might affect their sexual life. But most of spina bifida patients are fertile and are able to have children. Women born with open spina bifida should plan their pregnancy and are recommended to take 4 mg of folic acid a day (normal dose is 400 mcg) a month prior to conception and during early stages of pregnancy.

9.10 Cardiometabolic dysfunction

Patients with spina bifida affecting mobility have higher risk of developing components of metabolic syndrome in younger age due to low physical activity. They often suffer from abdominal obesity, insulin resistance or dyslipidemia with its metabolic and vascular complications [51]. People with physical disabilities spend less time performing physical activities compared to their nondisabled peers [52]. Consequences of a sedentary lifestyle include physical deconditioning [53]. Physical exercise can improve metabolic dysfunction [51].

Overweight, obesity, high BMI, high waist circumference and percentage of body fat are more prevalent in patients with spina bifida and they also have reduced aerobic fitness and muscle strenght [54]. Metabolic syndrome is more prevalent in spina bifida patients compared to nondisabled controls. They often display high levels of VLDL and overall cholesterol, triglycerides and low HDL, suffer from hypertension and insulin resistance [55].

Arterial diameters in these patients are reduced and sheer stress on the vascular wall is increased what predicts endothelial dysfunction [51].

9.11 Treatment of other complications

Patients with spina bifida often have post-operative complications, mainly infectious complications – wound and urinary infections, that require antibiotic therapy. According to frequent latex allergy in these patients, they should be operated and treated only in latex-free gloves in order to avoid severe anaphylactic reaction [11].

Special care must be taken to avoid pressure sores as due to lack of sensitivity and frequent hypomobility these patients are at higher risk of developing pressure sores and other wounds. All skin lesions in spina bifida have higher risk of getting infected.

Children with spina bifida often display precocious puberty and need to be examined by endocrinologist.

Due to frequent joint contractions, post-surgical immobilization and worse mobility these patients often suffer from osteoporosis and they are at higher risk of pathologic fractures. These fractures are more common in patients with higher level of neurological impairment due to more severe neurological deficit and this risk rises with age [11].

10. Prevention

As the effect of folic acid intake is known for its role in decreasing incidence of neural tube defects it has a great potential in prevention. Mandatory folic acid fortification has significantly higher effect on increasing serum folate levels that just recommendation [56]. Supplementation of folic acid starting at least one month prior conception and continuing through the first trimester of gravidity reduces the risk of neural tube defects. Because of the fact that many women discover their pregnancy within second months, what is late for prevention it is recommended for women in childbearing age to have long time daily supplement of 400 mcg of folic acid. Some foods such as: enriched bread, rice, cereals and pasta are fortified with 400 mcg of folic acid per serving. Except this also consumption of foods that are naturally rich in folate is recommended, such as: milk, egg yolks, avocado, citrus fruits and juices, beans and peas and dark green vegetables, as broccoli and spinach are.

Because of only available prevention of neural tube defects, that is also cheap and accessible, planned pregnancy is the best option. It is advised for women who plan pregnancy or are likely to get pregnant to have daily intake of 400 to 800 mcg of folic acid.

Fetal absorption of folic acid from mothers intake is better than absorption of folate from food. Combined with fact that most of the people do not have recommended intake of folate from diet rationale for intake of synthetic folic acid is high. There is an evidence, that proper intake of folic acid could lead to diminishing risk of also other developmental disorders – such as cleft lip, cleft palate and also congenital cardial defects. Women who were born with neural tube defect themselves or have anamnesis of birth or pregnancy with fetus with neural tube defect should take higher doses of folic acid. The same applies for women with anti-seizure medication.

11. Initial management

Management of treatment of severe forms of spina bifida that require surgical intervention begins just after diagnose. Prenatally diagnosed cases need to be referred to tertiary unit for further management. Usually first more detailed imagings are performed, genetic examination and screening for other congenital anomalies. Mothers with fetuses with spina bifida are referred to multidisciplinary team for pregnancy follow up, choosing the therapeutical strategy and timing of treatment in consensus with decision of instructed parents [23].

11.1 Delivery

All pregnancies with fetuses with more severe form of spina bifida are followed up in tertiary centres. Birth is usually scheduled from 38th week of gestation [23].

Babies with myelomeningocele tend to be in breech position. Breech position, cystic form of spinal defect or big sac are indications for ceasarian section. This type of delivery is also performed for its timing during the day when all specialists are available and newborn can be immediately treated.

11.2 Postpartal management

Directly after the birth newborn with open spinal defect is admitted to newborn intensive care unit and strictly monitored and stabilized. Newborns need to be properly examined for presence of other congenital defects or birth trauma, as well as evaluation of severity of spina bifida symptoms.

Examination of the newborn should include identification of level of paralysis of each extremity, presence of visible signs of spinal defect (skin lesion, visible sac), deformities of extremities (such a clubfoot, hip or knee contraction or dislocation) [11].

If newborn with open spinal defect did not underwent fetal surgery, postnatal surgery is indicated as soon as possible – just after stabilization of vital functions within the first days after delivery [46, 57]. Usually closure of spinal defect is indicated first with subsequent monitoring of ventricle size and symptoms of intracranial hypertension or symptoms of decompensation of Chiari malformation. Newborns who present with severe symptoms of intracranial hypertension at birth require shunt placement immediately.

Infants with stable slight ventricullomegaly with normal neurological status who are indicated for observation for hydrocephalus need to be routinely controlled. Clinical examination consists of evaluation of neurological status as well as regular frequent measurements of head circumference, palpation of fontanelle and cranial sutures. Also radiological controls are necessary. Best accessible is routine imaging of brain ventricles via head ultrasound and in special circumstances also use of magnetic resonance imaging.

After stabile postsurgical course with stable slight ventriculomegally and physiological neurological status with no symptoms of active hydrocephalus and decompensated Chiari II malformation, infant can be discharged to home with indication for frequent outpatient multidisciplinary evaluations. Weekly, later biweekly evaluations by neurosurgeon are necessary with active detection of symptoms of active hydrocephalus and decompensation of Chiari malformation. In some cases growth of head circumference will stabilize and follow normal growth curve and mild to moderate ventriculomegally will be stable.

Criteria for later indication of ventriculo-peritoneal shunting are onset of symptoms of intracranial hypertension (irritability, headache, somnolency, troubles with feeding, vomiting, bulging fontanelle, fixed downward gaze, „sunsetting "eye movements, bradycardia and sudden progress of head circumference), radiological finding of rapidly enlarged ventricles (via ultrasonography or MR imaging) and also worsening of Chiari II symptoms (abnormal eye movements, swallowing problems, apnoea or stridor). If these symptoms are present, infant should be immediately indicated for ventriculo-peritoneal drainage [58].

12. Follow up

Children with spina bifida, mostly open forms require very close follow up and observation for all possible problems. Most of the complications could be solved or at least properly managed to maintain adequate life quality. According to study with 50 years follow up 50% of patients born with myelomeningocele and surgically treated after birth were able to walk 50 m at the age of 9 years and 27% at the age of 50 years. Mobility decreases in time partially due to obesity and deterioration of general health conditions [22].

12.1 General practitioner

The role of **general practioner** – primary care doctor (pediatrician or family doctor) is very important. Doctor evaluates appropriate growth, indicates vaccination and general medical issues and coordinates medical care given by specialists. Patients and caregivers have to be properly instructed of the need of healthy life style, physical activity, precise monitoring of the skin status in order to prevent severe skin problems [59].

As most of patients with spina bifida thanks to advances in treatment reach adulthood there is a need for transition of health care to adult specialists [19]. Because the prevalence of obesity and metabolic syndrome is higher in these patients there is a need for careful monitoring of metabolic complications also in young patients [51].

Children and later also adult patients with diagnosis of open spina bifida after initial treatment need special treatment and follow up from various specialists:

12.2 Developmental pediatrician

This specialist should be part of the multidisciplinary team and survey the overall development of the child and indicate further examination of specialist when needed.

12.3 Neurosurgical controls

Child needs to be regularly controlled by neurosurgeon to evaluate proper function of ventriculoperitoneal drainage. Especially children with mild ventriculomegaly without symptoms of active hydrocephalus need regular controls so that in case symptoms develop could child immediately undergo surgery. Around half of the patients with open spinal defect undergoes other neurosurgical intervention in addition to initial spinal closure and half of these additional surgeries occur before 1 year of age – most common procedures are spinal closure, ventriculo-peritoneal shunt placement or shunt revision [38].

12.4 Neurology

All children after open neural tube defect with subsequent lasting neurological impairment need to be under supervision of experienced pediatric neurologist who controls motor functions, indexes progression of motor functions. In case of worsening of neurological functions there is a need for imaging – usually MR imaging for active screening of possible complications, such as tethered cord syndrome or decompensation of hydrocephalus, malfunction of drainage.

12.5 Urological controls

Each child after open spina bifida repair needs to be regularly evaluated by pediatric urologist. This evaluation consists of examination of kidney functions and urine derivation. Blood tests together with ultrasound and X-rays are often used, also other imaging techniques and urodynamic evaluation. Aim of this follow up is active screening for urological complications to prevent further damage. Since the survival of spina bifida patients has changed during years and most of patients live into adulthood there is also a need for management and follow up subsequently by adult urologist [24].

- Sexual health and education
- Gastroenterologist controls

12.6 Orthopedics and orthotics

The role of orthopedics is to monitor and treat deformities, follow up after early treatment, also monitor spinal balance and deformity and help in evaluation of motor function. The follow-up periodic orthopedical examination should include assessment of motor functions, sensitivity, range of motion, spinal deformity and integrity of skin. Early treatment of deformity by casting, bracing and surgical treatment may prevent fixed bony deformity [49].

Orthotics should periodically control the motor and mobility aids to ensure that orthoses are appropriate, in good shape and do not cause any pressure points on the skin [11].

12.7 Rehabilitation medicine and physical therapy

Special rehabilitations are necessary for children with open neural tube defect to increase movement, flexibility and muscle strenght. Skilled physical therapist plays an important role in the early detection of subtle muscle imbalance which could lead to severe deformity if left untreated. Therapist should perform serial manual muscle testing as a part of the routine at least annual examination [49].

There is a need for close cooperation between physical therapist and parents and caregivers to teach them basics of rehabilitation to practice it at home. For older children summer camps and recreational facilities for disabled are possibility to improve their physical activity. Some patients are also able to participate successfully in sports and should do so [51]. Basic physical strategies focus on muscle strengthening exercises, orthopedic supports and assistive devices meant to aid ambulation and posture control. Lifting weights is recommended for adolescents and adults to maintain condition of muscles. As patients have limited use of lower extremities, exercise has to rely on upper extremities and trunk. There is a potential for physical therapeutist to cooperate with local sport clubs and fitness centres to develop activity programs and supervise them [51]. Physical activities offer possibility to prevent other problems, such as obesity, metabolic problems or depression [52].

12.8 Psychologist and occupational therapy

Spina bifida patients have to face a lot of barriers to lead conventional life. As a result of physical disability, life-style, their environment and combination of these factors these patients are at higher risk of depressive disorder [60]. Teenagers, adolescents and also adults might feel isolated from their peers and have low self-esteem. They might feel worried, stressed, anxious or sad. If the feelings last for long time they might lead to depression. Occupational therapy and psychotherapy might help, as well as physical exercise. Daily physical activity is positively correlated with quality of life [51]. In serious cases consultation of psychiatrist might be necessary.

12.9 Neurocognitive rehabilitation

Many of children affected by open spina bifida, mostly those with implanted shunts to treat hydrocephalus have problems with concentration, hyperactivity, work slowly.

12.10 Special education teachers

Many children born with open spina bifida do not have problems at school. Children that present with some neurocognitive problems and special educational problems such as dyslexia or dyscalculia might profit from special education. Cognitive problems are more common in children who have hydrocephalus. Children at school need individualized educational plan with assistance. This plan is a result of cooperation of parents, teachers, school psychologist, school nurse and physical education teacher.

Patients with less severe forms of spinal dysraphism and lower level of spinal defect tend to reach higher educational effect. This is partially due to better mobility of these patients but very important factor is also bowel continence degree. Patients with bowel continence or sufficient incontinence control usually reach higher educational degrees, have higher employment and insurance status and are more likely to be independent, as educational status and employment are major determinants of health insurance status in adults [19]. Urinary incontinence does not have that impact on educational status as bowel incontinence. Bladder incontinence (particularly low-volume) has usually lower impact on overall life quality, educational status and employment than bowel incontinence [24, 48].

12.11 Social workers and social contact

There is an urgent need for adequate social contact of these children. Participation in sports and physical activity with peers improves social contact and life quality. Families can also contact Intervention programs for patients with spina bifida that work in many countries. Children with spina bifida meet a lot of barriers in acces to various activities and have to rely on adults to organize and supervise activities [51].

12.12 Dietitians

Proper diet is important to avoid complications mainly according to bowel function. With a help of dietitian can parents and caregivers find the best dietetic tools for each individual child. Addition of dietary fiber can help to maintain regular stool. Enough water intake is important in prevention of obstipation and urinary infection. Proper dietary intake together with physical exercise helps to prevent overweight and obesity that could lead to metabolic syndrome and cause later metabolic and cardiovascular complications [51].

13. Prognosis

In the 1950s the survival rate of patients with most severe form of spina bifida – myelomeningocele was about 10% [61]. In the last decades, the multidisciplinary approach to care of spina bifida patients, has significantly improved patients outcomes. Recently, thanks to advances in medical and supporting treatment almost all children born with spina bifida survive into adulthood. There has been increase in life expectancy and gain in the quality of life of spina bifida patients but also of their caregiver's life [43] But unfortunately, neurological outcomes of spina bifida patients did not change significantly over the years of medical progress [44]. That is mostly due to fact, that the neurological impairment is mostly caused by primary damage from congenital spinal abnormality and also secondary due to exposure of nervous tissue to amniotic fluid [21].

Important factor for prognosis is ability to attain early ambulation. It provides physiological and psychological benefits even if the child will later become a sitter. Also patients with high-level spina bifida who participated in walking program have lower risk of fractures, pressure sores are more independent than those who had been prescribed wheelchair early [11].

According to long term follow up study median survival of myelomeningocele patients was 50 years. 34% of patients had died before 5 years of age. Most common cause of death was cardiorespiratory, neurological and urological complications, then hydrocephalus and infections of central nervous system, other causes are significantly less frequent [22].

Most of the survivors had IQ over 80 points. Only one fifth was fully continent without need of incontinency aids. One third of patients recorded chronic back pain.

Percentage of patients living independently on their caregivers raises in time after age of 25. Independent living at the age of 50 years is more common in patients without anamnesis of intracranial hypertension and without cerebrospinal fluid shunt revisions [22]. Increase of independent living with age might be partially due to fact that longer survival is associated with less severe primary defect.

14. Conclusion

Spina bifida occulta is usually an incidental finding with no effect on life quality. On the other hand, the most severe form myelomeningocele is a complex problem. Due to many complications threatening patient with this complex health issue, there is an essential need for multidisciplinary approach to monitor, prevent and treat possible complications that have impact on functionality, life quality and survival. Parents and close caregivers have crucial role in whole mutidisciplinary team. They need to know how to manage child's situation and give child social and emotional support. Raising the child in caring environment could help to develop into young adult who is able to fight basic life issues: to care about his own health issues, going to school, working, finding and using transportation, living in their own and having a healthy relationship and family.

Author details

Romana Richterová*, Branislav Kolarovszki and René Opšenák
Clinic of Neurosurgery, Jessenius Faculty of Medicine of Commenius University in Bratislava, University Hospital in Martin, Martin, Slovakia

*Address all correspondence to: romana.richterova@gmail.com

References

[1] Sewell MJ, Chiu YE, Drolet BA (2015) Neural tube dysraphism: review of cutaneous markers and imaging. Pediatr Dermatol 32:161-170. https ://doi.org/ 10.1111/pde.12485

[2] Ben-Sira L, Ponger P, Miller E, Beni-Adani L, Constantini S (2009) Low-risk lumbar skin stigmata in infants: the role of ultrasound screening. J Pediatr 155:864-869. https ://doi. org/10.1016/j. jpeds .2009.06.003

[3] Valente I, Pedicelli A, Piacentini M, Di Serafino M, Vallone G, Speca S, Colosimo C.J Spinal cord ultrasonography of the newborn. Ultrasound. 2019 Jun;22(2):113-119. doi: 10.1007/s40477-018-0345-y. Epub 2018 Dec 7.

[4] Meyers AB, Chandra T, Epelman M (2017) Sonographic spinal imaging of normal anatomy, pathology and magnetic growing rods in children. Pediatr Radiol 47:1046-1057. https ://doi. org/10.1007/s0024 7-017-3845-6 .

[5] Schwartz ES, Rossi A (2015) Congenital spine anomalies: the closed spinal dysraphisms. Pediatr Radiol 45:413-419. https ://doi.org/10.1007/ s0024 7-015-3425-6

[6] Au K.S., Ashley-Koch A., Northrup H. Epidemiologic and genetic aspects of spina bifida and other neural tube defects. Dev Disabil Res Rev. 2010;16(1):6-15. doi: 10.1002/ddrr.93.

[7] Morton CC, Metcalfe A, Kamran Y, Sibbald B,Wilson RD. The Impact of Prenatal Diagnosis of Selected Central Nervous System Anomalies for Prenatal Counseling Based on Significant Pregnancy Morbidity and Neonatal Outcomes. J Obstet Gynaecol Can, 2019 Feb; 41(2): 166-173. e1. doi: 10.1016/j.jogc

[8] Bodin CR, Rasmussen MM, Tabor A, Westbom L, Tiblad E, Ekelund CK, Wulff CB, Vogel I, Petersen OB. Ultrasound in prenatal diagnostics and its impact on the epidemiology of spina bifida in a national cohort from Denmark with a comparison to Sweden. Biomed Res Int 2018; **2018**: 9203985.

[9] Atta CAM, Fiest KM, Frolkis AD, et al. Global birth prevalence of spina bifida by folic acid forti fi cation status : A systematic review and meta- analysis. 2016;106. DOI: 10.2105/AJPH.2015. 302902

[10] Yi Y, Lindemann M, Colligs A, Snowball C. Economic burden of neural tube defects and impact of prevention with folic acid: a literature review. Eur J Pediatr. 2011;170(11):1391-1400

[11] Swaroop VT, Dias L. Orthopedic management of spina bifida. Part I: hip, knee, and rotational deformities. J Child Orthop. 2009 Dec;3(6):441-9. doi: 10.1007/s11832-009-0214-5. Epub 2009 Oct 25.PMID: 19856195

[12] Choi JH, Lee T, Kwon HH, You SK, Kang JW. Outcome of ultrasonographic imaging in infants with sacral dimple. Korean J Pediatr. 2018 Jun;61(6):194-199. doi: 10.3345/kjp.2018.61.6.194. Epub 2018 Jun 25.

[13] Sarikaya Solak S, Kivanc Altunay I, Tukenmez Demirci G, Can B. Prevalence of congenital cutaneous anomalies in 1000 newborns and a review of the literature. Am J Perinatol 2016;33:79-83.

[14] Irani N, Goud AR, Lowe LH. Isolated filar cyst on lumbar spine sonography in infants: a case-control study. Pediatr Radiol 2006;36: 1283-1288.

[15] Kucera JN, Coley I, O'Hara S, Kosnik EJ, Coley BD (2014) The simple sacral dimple: diagnostic yield of ultrasound in neonates. Pediatr Radiol 45:211-216. https ://doi.org/10.1007/ s0024 7-014-3110-1

[16] Zywicke HA, Rozzelle CJ (2011) Sacral Dimples. Pediatr Rev 32:109-114. https ://doi.org/10.1542/pir.32-3-109

[17] Chern JJ, Kirkman JL, Shannon CN, Tubbs RS, Stone JD, Royal SA, et al. Use of lumbar ultrasonography to detect occult spinal dysraphism clinical article. J Neurosur Pediatr 2012;9:274-279.

[18] Dicianno B.E., Karmarkar A., Houtrow A. et al. Factors associated with mobility outcomes in a national spina bifida patient registry. Am J Phys Med Rehabil 2015; 94:1015-1025.

[19] Swank M, Dias LS (1994) Walking ability in spina bifida patients: a model for predicting future ambulatory status based on sitting balance and motor level. J Pediatr Orthop 14:715-718

[20] Wiener JS, Suson KD, Castillo J, Routh JC, Tanaka S, Liu T, Ward E, Thibadeau J, Joseph D, Registry NSBP. Bowel management and continence in adults with spina bifida: Results from the National Spina Bifida Patient Registry 2009-15. J Pediatr Rehabil Med. 2017 Dec 11;10(3-4):335-343. doi: 10.3233/PRM-170466.

[21] Adzick NS. Fetal surgery for spina bifida: past, present, future. Semin Pediatr Surg 2013; 22: 10-17.

[22] Oakeshott P., Poulton A., Hunt G. M., Reid F. Walking and living independently with spina bifida: a 50-year prospective cohort study. Dev Med Child Neurol . 2019 Oct;61(10):1202-1207. doi: 10.1111/dmcn.14168. Epub 2019 Jan 23.

[23] Sileo, F.G., Pateisky, P., Curado, J., Evans, K., Hettige, S., Thilaganathan, B. Long-term neuroimaging and neurological outcome of fetal spina bifida aperta after postnatal surgical repair. Ultrasound Obstet Gynecol 2019; 53: 309-313. DOI: 10.1002/uog.20215

[24] Wiener JS, Suson KD, Castillo J, Routh JC, Tanaka ST, Liu T, Ward EA, Thibadeau JK, Joseph DB; National Spina Bifida Patient Registry. Bladder Management and Continence Outcomes in Adults with Spina Bifida: Results from the National Spina Bifida s, 2009 to 2015. J Urol. 2018 Jul;200(1):187-194. doi: 10.1016/j.juro.2018.02.3101. Epub 2018 Mar 26.PMID: 29588216

[25] Rocque BG, Bishop ER, Scogin MA, et al. Assessing health-related quality of life in children with spina bifida. Journal of Neurosurgery: Pediatrics 2015; 15(2): 144. [PubMed: 25415252]

[26] Norkett W, McLone DG, Bowman R. Current Management Strategies of Hydrocephalus in the Child With Open Spina Bifida.Top Spinal Cord Inj Rehabil. 2016 Fall;22(4):241-246. doi: 10.1310/sci2204-241.PMID: 29339864

[27] Rekate HL. The definition and classification of hydrocephalus: a personal recommendation to stimulate debate. Cerebrospinal Fluid Res. 2008; 5:2. [PubMed: 18211712]

[28] Tully HM, Dobyns WB. Infantile hydrocephalus: a review of epidemiology, classification and causes. Eur J Med Genet. 2014 Aug;57(8):359-68. doi: 10.1016/j.ejmg.2014.06.002. Epub 2014 Jun 13.PMID: 24932902

[29] Tamburrini G, Frassanito P, Iakovaki K, et al. Myelomeningocele: The management of the associated hydrocephalus. Childs Nerv Syst. 2013;29(9):1569-1579.

[30] Adzick N, Thom EA, Spong CY, et al; MOMS Investigators. A randomized trial of prenatal versus postnatal repair of myelomeningocele. New Engl J Med. 2011;364(11):993-1004.

[31] Sweeney KJ, et al. Spinal level of myelomeningocele lesion as a contributing factor in posterior fossa volume, intracranial cerebellar volume, and cerebellar ectopia. J Neurosurg Pediatr. 2013; 11(2):154-159. [PubMed: 23157392]

[32] Hertzler DA 2nd, DePowell JJ, Stevenson CB, et al. Tethered cord syndrome: a review of the literature from embryology to adult presentation. Neurosurg Focus. 2010;29(1):E1.

[33] Catmull S, Ashurst J. Tethered Cord Syndrome. Clin Pract Cases Emerg Med. 2019 Jul 3;3(3):297-298. doi: 10.5811/cpcem.2019.4.42536. eCollection 2019 Aug.

[34] Chao TT, Dashe JS, Adams RC, et al. Fetal spine findings on MRI and associated outcomes in children with open neural tube defects. AJR Am J Roentgenol 2011;197:956-61 CrossRef Medline

[35] Sullivan PB. Gastrointestinal disorders in children with neurodevelopmental disabilities. Dev Disabil Res Rev 2008; 14:128-136

[36] Patel, J., Walker, J.L., Talwalkar, V.R., Iwinski, H.J., Milbrandt, T.A. Correlation of spine deformity, lung function, and seat pressure in spina bifida. Clin Orthop Relat Res. 2011 May;469(5):1302-1307. doi: 10.1007/s11999-010-1687-8.

[37] Copp AJ, Adzick NS, Chitty LS, Fletcher JM, Holmbeck GN, Shaw GM. Spina bifida. Nat Rev Dis Primers. 2015 Apr 30;1:15007. doi: 10.1038/nrdp.2015.7.

[38] Alabi, N.B, Thibadeau J., Wiener, J.S., Conklin, M.J., Dias, M.S., Sawin, K.J., Valdez, R. Surgeries and Health Outcomes Among Patients With Spina Bifida. Pediatrics 2018 Sep;142(3):e20173730. doi: 10.1542/peds.2017-3730.

[39] Committee on Obstetric Practice Society for Maternal-Fetal Medicine. Maternal-fetalsurgeryformyelomeningocele.2017;130:164-67Medline

[40] Nagaraj U.D., Bierbrauer K.S., Stevenson C.B., Peiro J.L, Lim F.Y. Spinal Imaging Findings of Open Spinal Dysraphisms on Fetal and Postnatal MRI AJNR Am J Neuroradiol. 2018 Oct;39(10):1947-1952. doi: 10.3174/ajnr.A5760. Epub 2018 Sep 20.

[41] Ausili E, Maresca G, Massimi L, Morgante L, Romagnoli C, Rendeli C (2018) Occult spinal dysraphisms in newborns with skin markers: role of ultrasonography and magnetic resonance imaging. Child's Nerv Syst 34:285-291. https ://doi.org/10.1007/s0038 1-017-3638-0

[42] Cerovac A, Serak A, Zukic H, Nevacinovic E, Ljuca D, Brigic A, Habek D. Ethical and Legal Dilemmas Around Termination of Pregnancy for Severe Fetal Hydrocephalus, Spina Bifida Aperta and Meningomyelocoella. Med Arch. 2019 Apr;73(2):126-130. doi: 10.5455/medarh.2019.73.126-130.

[43] Snow-Lisy DC, Yerkes EB, Cheng EY. Update on urological management of spina bifida from prenatal diagnosis to adulthood. J Urol 2015; 194: 288.

[44] North T, Cheong A, Steinbok P, Radic JA. Trends in incidence and long-term outcomes of myelomeningocele in British Columbia. Childs Nerv Syst 2018; 34: 717-724.

[45] Zarutskie A, Guimaraes C, Yepez M, Torres P, Shetty A, Sangi-Haghpeykar H, Lee W, Espinoza J, Shamshirsaz AA, Nassr A, Belfort MA, Whitehead WE, Sanz Cortes M. Prenatal brain imaging for predicting need for postnatal hydrocephalus treatment in fetuses that had neural tube defect repair in utero. Ultrasound Obstet Gynecol. 2019 Mar;53(3):324-334. doi: 10.1002/uog.20212.

[46] Attenello FJ, Tuchman A, Christian EA, Wen T, Chang KE, Nallapa S, Cen SY, Mack WJ, Krieger MD, McComb JG. Infection rate correlated with time to repair of open neural tube defects (myelomeningoceles): an institutional and national study. Childs Nerv Syst 2016; **32**: 1675-1681.

[47] Inversetti A, Van Der Veeken L, Thompson D, Jansen K, Van Calenbergh F, Joyeux L, Bosteels J, Deprest J. Neurodevelopmental outcome of children with spina bifida aperta repaired prenatally *vs* postnatally: systematic review and meta-analysis. Ultrasound Obstet Gynecol 2019; **53**: 293-301.

[48] Szymanski KM, Cain MP, Whittam B, et al. All incontinence is not created equal: impact of urinary and fecal incontinence on quality of life in adults with spina bifida. J. Urol 2017; 197(3): 885. [PubMed: 28131501]

[49] Swaroop VT, Dias L. Orthopaedic management of spina bifida-part II: foot and ankle deformities.J Child Orthop. 2011 Dec;5(6):403-14. doi: 10.1007/s11832-011-0368-9. Epub 2011 Sep 20.PMID: 23205142

[50] Akbar M, Bresch B, Seyler TM, Wenz W, Bruckner T, Abel R, Carstens C (2009) Management of orthopaedic sequelae of congenital spinal disorders. J Bone Joint Surg Am 91:87-100

[51] Short KR, Frimberger D. A review of the potential for cardiometabolic dysfunction in youth with spina bifida and the role for physical activity and structured exercise. Int J Pediatr. 2012; 2012:541363. doi: 10.1155/2012/541363.

[52] Claridge, E.A., Bloemen' M.A.T., Rook, R.A, Obeid, J., Timmons, B.W., Takken, T., Van Den Berg-Emons, R. J. G, De Groot, J.F., Gorter, J.W. Physical activity and sedentary behaviour in children with spina bifida. Dev Med Child Neurol. 2019 Dec;61(12):1400-1407. doi: 10.1111/dmcn.14333. Epub 2019 Aug 30.

[53] Rimmer, J. H., Schiller, W. and Chen M.D. "Effects of disability-associated low energy expenditure deconditioning syndrome," Exercise and Sport Sciences Reviews, vol. 40, no. 1, pp. 22-29, 2012.

[54] Schoenmakers, M. A. G. C., de Groot, J. F. , Gorter, J. W., Hillaert, J. L. M., Helders, P. J. M. and Takken, T. "Muscle strength, aerobic capacity and physical activity in independent ambulating children with lumbosacral spina bifida," Disability and Rehabilitation, vol. 31, no. 4, pp. 259-266, 2009.

[55] Nelson, M. D. , Widman, L. M., Abresch R. T. et al., "Metabolic syndrome in adolescents with spinal cord dysfunction," Journal of Spinal Cord Medicine, vol. 30, no. 1, pp. S127–S139, 2007.

[56] Herrmann W, Obeid R. Themandatoryfortificationof staple foods with folic acid: a current controversy in Germany. Dtsch Arztebl Int. 2011;108(15):249-254.

[57] Mattogno PP, Massimi L, Tamburrini G, Frassanito P, Di Rocco C, Caldarelli M. Myelomeningocele repair: surgical management based on a 30-year experience. Acta Neurochir Suppl 2017; **124**: 143-148.

[58] Chakraborty A, Crimmins D, Hayward R, et al. Toward reducing shunt placement rates in patients with myelomeningocele. J Neurosurg Pediatr. 2008;1:361-365.

[59] Thibadeau, J, Walker Jr, W.O, Castillo, J., Dicianno, B.E., Routh, J.C, Smith, K.A., Ouyang, L. Philosophy of care delivery for spina bifida. Disabil Health J. 2020 Apr;13(2):100883. doi: 10.1016/j.dhjo.2019.100883.

[60] Bloemen MAT, Backx FJG, Takken T, et al. Factors associated with physical activity in children and adolescents with a physical disability: a systematic review. Dev Med Child Neurol 2015; 57: 137-148

[61] Laurence K. Effect of early surgery for spina bifida on survival and quality of life. Lancet. 1974;1:301-304

Chapter 3

Surgical Treatment of Neural Tube Defects

Juraj Šutovský

Abstract

Neural tube defects (NTDs) are developmental pathologies associated with undesirable lifelong consequences. Incidence of these pathologies differs between countries and regions depending on socio-economic and healthcare quality. It is also influenced by folic acid and zinc supplementation. Genetic factors influence probability of NTD, increasing risk of defect in siblings up to 3–8%. Estimated incidence in United States is 3–4/10000 live births, and worldwide incidence increases on about 10/10000 live births. Despite various types and localizations of spina bifida, in all of them neural tissue is in danger. This can lead to various types of neurologic disorders. Not only due to direct damaging of spinal cord and nerve roots but also other parts of central nervous system are also endangered by disturbed prenatal development. Other consequences as orthopedic abnormalities, bladder, and bowel dysfunction influence quality of life. Surgical therapy is often the only possibility to preserve existing function of neural tissue, allows its further development and prevents complications. In this chapter surgical techniques with aim to restore spinal cord and nerve roots anatomy, preservation of its function and defect closures are presented. Also, treatment of possible comorbidities and complications is discussed. Spina bifida management requires multi-speciality cooperation and care to monitor, prevent and treat various potential complication that can negatively influence quality of life and even survival. Prenatal diagnosis is based on maternal screening of serum alpha fetoprotein (AFP) levels and prenatal ultrasonography examination. As the suspicion of neural tube defect arises, an amniocentesis is recommended to complete a genetic analysis and obtain amniotic fluid for more precise AFP and acetylcholinesterase examination. Some types of neural tube defects are diagnosed after delivery, some are symptomatic until adulthood and some are diagnosed incidentally. Each of them requires specific management, based on underlying pathology.

Keywords: neural tube defect, neural placode, spina bifida, hydrocephalus, tethered spinal cord

1. Introduction

Neural tube defect is with congenital heart defect the most serious birth anomaly compatible with life. Besides genetic influences, zinc and folic acid deficiency plays important role [1]. As neural tube closure occurs in fourth gestation week its failure should be diagnosed early during pregnancy. Despite spontaneous defect closure had been reported [2], once neural tube defect is diagnosed a pregnancy termination is an option. Up to 60% diagnosed NTS in Europe ends with planned termination of pregnancy [3].

Another option is in utero surgery, open or fetoscopic.

In the case of late diagnosis or gravidity does not match prenatal surgery criteria or just because in utero surgery is not accessible, postnatal surgery comes in role.

If spina bifida is diagnosed prenatally, delivery should be done in center with capabilities for taking care for both, mother, and new-born.

2. Spina bifida

Spina bifida aperta

Myelomeningocele

Myelomeningocele is the most common type of spina bifida aperta resulting in defective neural tube closure between 22nd and 26th days of gestation. Most occurred at lower lumbar segment, with neurological impairment below level of lesion. Not only distorted development but also exposure to amniotic fluid, toxic to neural tissue, is the cause of neural tissue malfunction.

In this type of spina bifida aperta, unclosed neural tube, neural placode is exposed directly to external environment and through arachnoid/connective tissue is attached to dysplastic skin (**Figure 1**).

Almost all cases are associated with some degree of Chiari ll. malformation, and majority of them requires CSF derivation due to hydrocephalus.

Preoperative management

Because neural tissue in spina bifida aperta/myelomeningocele is exposed to external environment delivery is planned as cesarean delivery to minimize risk of infection. Nonlatex gloves usage is recommended while handling a baby due to possible allergy. Immediately after delivery, the open spina bifida must be covered with a sterile non-adherent saline-soaked dressing to prevent infection and dehydration due to CSF and interstitial fluid losses.

Postnatal thorough examination is recommended to rule out other congenital malformations and conditions that prevent early surgery, especially pulmonary and cardiac malformations. Cranial ultrasound is obligatory for cranial malformation identification. Preoperative MRI is helpful for anatomical orientation and associated pathology exclusion (**Figure 2**). If there are no contraindications, operation is indicated as soon as possible ideally up to 12 hours postnatally but not more than 24 hours. Any delay in spina bifida closure increases risk of infection and hemodynamic instability.

Besides early surgery, broad spectrum antibiotics are warranted administered, at least until the skin lesion is closed, to minimize the risk of infection of the central nervous system.

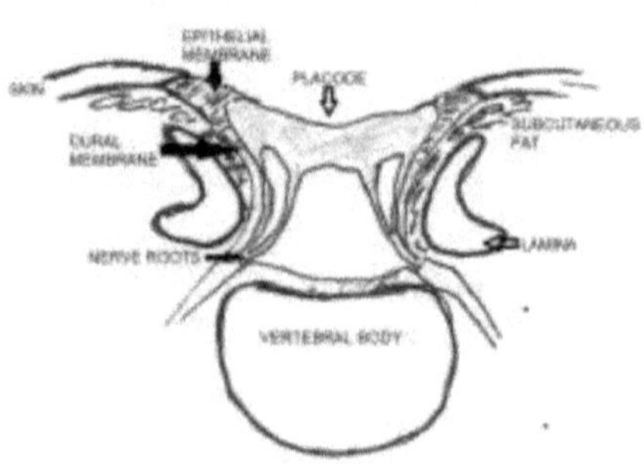

Figure 1.
Schematic picture of myelomeningocele. Neural placode is in direct contact with external environment.

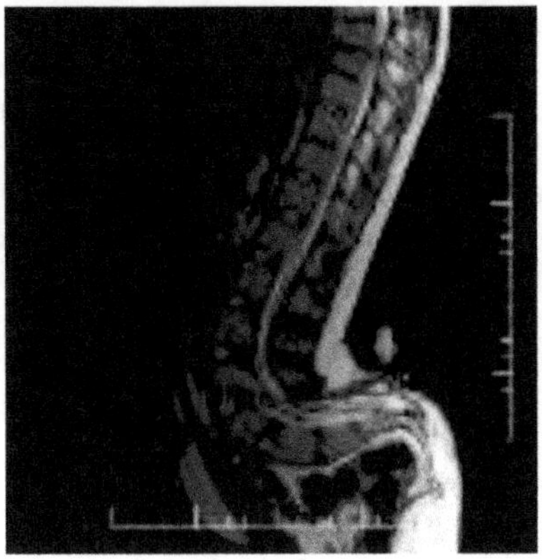

Figure 2.
Sacral myelomeningocele (red arrow) on T2 MRI.

At the surgical theater new-born should be positioned prone or laterally to avoid pressure on the placode prior to surgery. Besides dehydration attention must be paid to possible hypothermia.

Before operation field preparation swabs for aerobic and anaerobic cultures should be taken.

Because of exposed neural tissue, operation field is prepared only with sterile saline and surrounding skin can be prepared in standard manner. Draping must be adapted to planned type of surgery. If direct closure of skin defect is in question, sufficient visible skin must be left for flap reconstruction. Swabs for aerobic and anaerobic cultures should be taken form the skin and CSF samples as soon as CSF is encountered.

Neural tube closure

Spina bifida surgery must be done under microscopic control. Sharp dissection is mandatory to prevent traction injury to already damaged neural tissue. The primal incision starts in midline cranially to the lesion, best above the level of identified spinous process cranial to defect. Dissection continues caudally to the placode at the border between skin and arachnoid, which is not regular with possible extension of dystrophic skin reaching placode. Cranial view from upper part of the placode reveals spinal cord emerging from the spinal canal. Separation of neural placode with adjacent arachnoid continues in step by step manner. After circumferential neural placode dissection from skin, all arachnoid adhesions must be released, preventing spinal cord tethering. Dissection must be done with awareness of possible spinal nerves lateral to placode adherent to sac.

After deliberation thorough inspection of neural placode must be done to remove any non-nerve tissue reducing not only possibility of future spinal cord tethering but also preventing epidermoid/dermoid cyst or lipoma formation. In cases of lipomyelomeningocele, with indistinct boundaries between neural and adipose tissue, perioperative neuromonitoring is useful and should be used.

Dorsal nerve roots usually just below placode edge and ventral roots emerging more medially from the ventral side of placode are inspected and are released from adhesions allowing neural tube reconstruction without tension. Aberrant nerve roots ending blindly in dura must be divided.

At the caudal end of placode filum terminale should be identified. When it is clearly recognizable, its section is indicated to minimize risk of tethered spinal cord and prevent future neurological deterioration and need for another operation.

During surgery not only neural tissue but also vascular supply must be managed carefully. Vessels passing from formed spinal cord and nerve root vessels must be preserved. If any bleeding occurs, avoiding coagulation is recommended until inevitable. Primal management of bleeding can be done with haemostatic material (Gelaspon or Flo-seal) or cotton patches alone.

After placode deliberation inspection for any other fixation point is mandatory (**Figure 3**). The attempt to reconstruct neural tube is the next step. Approximation of lateral edges medially with arachnoid-pial sutures partially re-create tubular spinal cord with arachnoid-pial outer surface, what minimizes risk of adhesions and spinal cord fixation. Non-absorbable 7/0 – 8/0 monofilament sutures are used. Care must be taken not to "squeeze" neural tissue with sutures. If the placode is too bulky relinquish attempt to reconstruct neural tube not to damage liveable neural tissue at the cost of higher possibility of spinal cord tethering.

After the placode is released and neural tube is reconstructed eventually, dural sac closure is the next step.

Intact dura is identified at the cranial part of defect, at the site of lower lamina. After dura is identified at the upper part, epidural fat and space between vertebral structures and dura is the plane for sharp dissection and identification of dural lateral borders, where dura continuously passes to the thoracolumbar fascia. At this transition, dura must be divided by sharp dissection. If there is a sufficient dura for primary closure of dural sac without neural tissue compression, dura is closed with continuous suture with non-absorbable 5/0 monofilament thread. If there is no sufficient dural covering for closure or closure without compression of neural tissue, grafts must be used. As a first choice is autologous substitute harvested from thoracolumbar fascia or muscular flap from latissimus dorsi muscle. If there is no possibility acquiring sufficient autologous flap, nowadays artificial collagen substitute of dura (DuraGen) can be used. Attention must be paid to eliminate any compression of neural tissue, allowing free passage of CSF around deliberated placode and prevent later adhesion.

If there is any suspicion of possible CSF leakage, dural glue helps to prevent complication. Eventually another layer formed by thoracolumbar fascia can be added if there is enough material left. Vertical parallel fascial incisions help mobilization of thoracolumbar fascia (**Figure 4**).

Skin closure

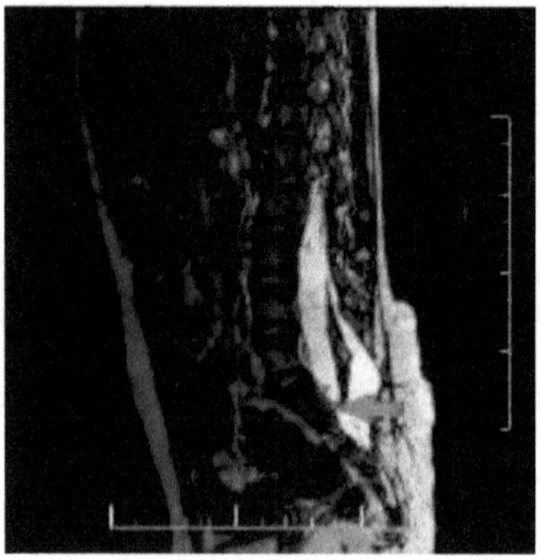

Figure 3.
Thickened filum terminale (red arrow) fixing spinal cord after successful myelomeningocele reconstruction.

Direct suture in small defects is most often doable. Undermining skin laterally helps relax tension on suture. Absorbable adaptational subcutaneous sutures help to relieve strain on skin edges, eventually subcutaneous tissue can be fixed to medial thoracolumbar fascia. Skin is closed with non-absorbable 5/0 monofilament. If there is still tension on the skin suture, lateral longitudinal relaxing incisions in the similar manner as the thoracolumbar fascia relaxation, without reaching subcutaneous tissue.

If a direct suture is impossible, cutaneous flap can be used to release tension on the suture. Usage of flap type depends on defect localization and surgeon's familiarity with surgical technique. A single rotational flap is the simplest one. The universal rhomboid (Limberg) flap useful in closure bigger defects. Also, O-to-Z flap can be helpful in skin closure especially in more longitudinal than wide defects (**Figure 5**).

If neurosurgeon is not completely familiar with skin flap techniques, or skin defect is too large, plastic surgeon should be a part of surgical team.

Postoperative management

After skin closure operative field is disinfected in standard manner and wound is covered with sterile non-adhesive covering (Atrauman, Atrauman Ag) to prevent wound injury during redressing, and sterile gauze. To prevent wound contamination postoperatively with urine and stool, wound is covered with plastic adhesive drape.

Postoperatively prone position with pelvis little bit elevated, to release CSF pressure in lumbar region. Prone position is preferred up to 7th postoperative day.

Wide spectrum intravenous prophylactic antibiotics are indicated at least 24 hours postoperatively. Better choice is extended prophylaxis until results from perioperatively samples are negative. If cultivation reveals infection, therapeutic regimen according results is indicated.

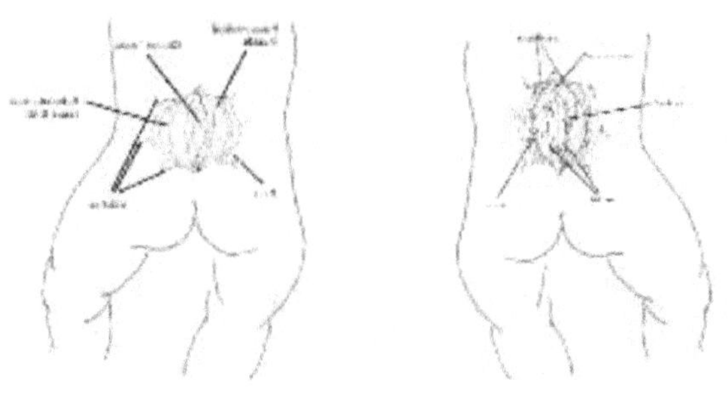

Figure 4.
After dural closure, with, or without graft, curvilinear fascial incision is helpful in thoracolumbar fascia mobilization and addition another covering layer.

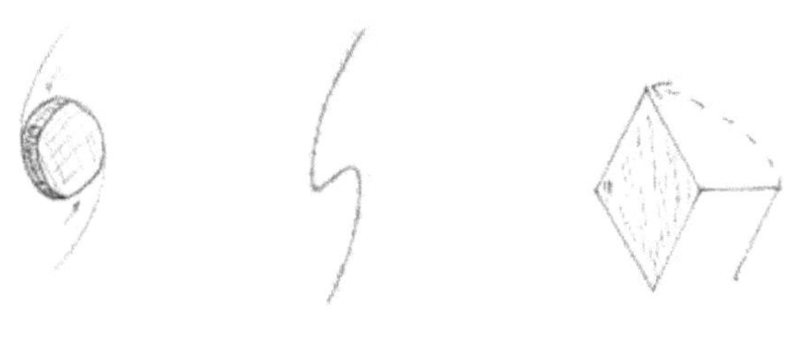

Figure 5.
Skin closure usually possible with direct suture. In cases of larger defects, O-to-Z, or Limberg flaps are helpful in releasing suture tension.

Early postoperative complications

Due to exposure of neural tissue to outer environment, insufficient skin coverage, stress due to pain, surgical procedure and feeding problems, complication related to wound healing occurs.

Most common is skin healing problem. It is often due to insufficient blood supply because of high tension at the suture site or extended skin undermining with perforator vessel damaging. Usually skin necrosis is only superficial and besides daily check-up does not need any other action and reepithelization occurs. If the skin is affected in full thickness with deeper layer consisting of thoracolumbar fascia with underlying muscles are intact, debridement of necrotic tissue must be done until normal tissue with blood oozing from edges is apparent. With no other complication secondary healing with reepithelization from edges occurs, despite it takes longer time and meticulous wound management preventing secondary infection is necessary. Necrosis whole thickness of reconstructed dura covering requires revision surgery with plastic surgeon to recover defect with sufficiently vascularized flap.

After surgery wound must be inspected on daily basis to identify any problem with wound healing. Any collection under the skin worsen healing applying tension to the wound. The cause of tension and collection must be identified by aspiration. Hematoma or interstitial fluid collection must be evacuated. Not only internal, but also external compression from wound dressing must be avoided.

If there is CSF collection, just on 1st-3rd day after surgery with no apparent progression and tension, it may be due to fragile lumbar dura, CSF oozes around the stitches and collection resolves spontaneously up to 6th–7th day after surgery. Closure of dural defect can lead to changes in CSF flow pattern, with increasing pressure in subarachnoid and intraventricular spaces. In this case CSF may accumulate at the surgical site later, usually on 5th–7th day after surgery. If there are no sign of progressive hydrocephalus and closure is done in standard manner, collection may dissipate spontaneously after subarachnoid/intraventricular pressure comes to balance.

With any doubts or problems about the sufficient closure of all layers with progressive cumulation of subcutaneous CSF collection even if there is CSF leakage through the skin suture, CSF derivation and surgery site revision is indicated.

External ventricular drain, despite higher risk of neuroinfection, or subcutaneous reservoir (Rickham, Omaya) is the first option in cases without hydrocephalus. It is necessary keep in mind, that reservoir is associated with need for repeatedly evacuations of CSF what increases risk of infection and is also painful and stressful procedure.

Ventriculoperitoneal shunt in the case of CSF leak at the site of spina bifida closure is not ideal option, because valve opening pressure is usually higher as the pressure of sutured soft tissues at the site of spina bifida, thus not solve the problem. Possibility is the programmable valve with adjusted opening pressure on 0 mm Hg and after resolution wound problem readjusted to the desired level.

Surgical site infection is relatively rare. Reported incidence is about 1–12% [4].

If the wound infection is identified, without signs of intradural infection, and no presence of any subcutaneous collection, swabs for microbiological examination from surgical site should be done and local therapy applied. If there are signs of abscess formation, aspiration of purulent material for aerobic and anaerobic cultivation should be obtained and releasing of few sutures for effective drainage and antimicrobial rinsing abscess cavity. Wound defect is left for secondary intention.

If there are signs of neuraxis infection proved by clinical and laboratory examination, CNS penetrating wide spectrum antibiotics are administered. After cultivation proves infection, targeted antibiotics are indicated. In any suspicion of surgical site intradural infection, revision is indicated with removing of purulent content avoiding placode and nerve roots damage with surgical site irrigation with antibiotic solution. Wound reclosure in done in the same manner as in the primary surgery.

Meningocele

Meningocele is another open neural tube defect with protruding only meninges through the insufficient lamina and back soft tissue. Neural structures are not a part of the sac. Sometimes meninges are not fully visible from the outside but are covered with dysplastic or fully developed skin. As there is no damage to the neural structures, long time outcome is more favorable as is in myelomeningocele.

Prenatal, postnatal, and surgical management is identical to myelomeningocele with no necessity of neural tube reconstruction.

Because there is s malformation of dural development, during surgery is warranted close inspection of spinal cord with releasing it from any possible arachnoideal, fibrous adhesion to prevent from tethered spinal cord. Also, filum terminale should inspected and cut if it is in the surgical field [5].

Prenatal surgery

Prenatal surgery is an option in OSB cases. According to MOMS study (Management of Myelomeningocele Study) foetal surgery [6] is promising treatment which reduce need for VPS approximately of 50% and lower incidence of severe hindbrain herniation and improve ability to walk independently (**Figure 6**).

But according to metanalysis study, prenatal spinal closure does not reduce the possibility of SCT, conversely higher incidence is reported [7] (**Figure 7**).

This result must be evaluating with caution because foetal surgery is demanding procedure associated with risk of premature birth, potential morbidity for mother and can be limitation for further pregnancies.

Spina bifida occulta

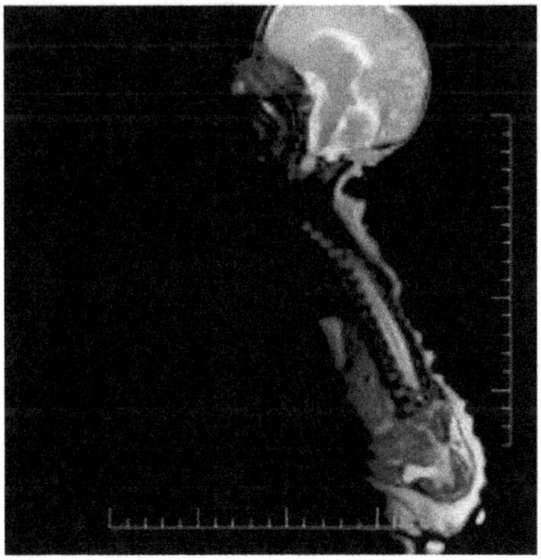

Figure 6.
Complete resolution (red arrow) of hindbrain herniation after in utero myelomeningocele closure.

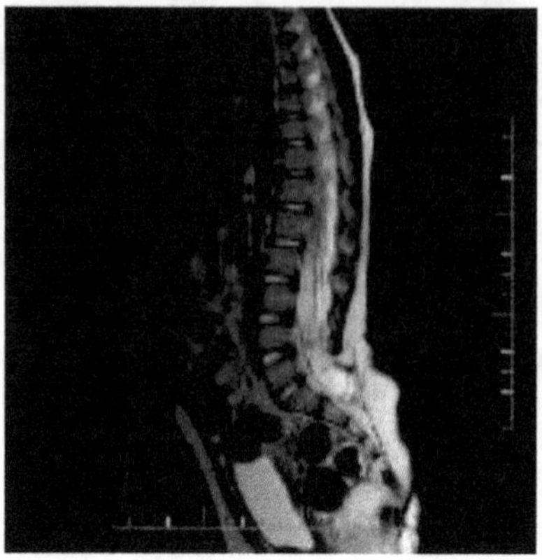

Figure 7.
Despite prenatal surgery, tethered spinal cord persist postnatally.

Many defects of neural tube closure are not apparent, so they are named "spina bifida occulta" (SBO) or "closed spina bifida". As these defects are results of failed secondary neurulation, they are covered with continuous, sufficient skin.

There are several subtypes of SBO. Cystic lesion protruding through open spinal canal covered with sufficient skin can be formed only with meninges – meningocele, containing only fat tissue – lipomeningocele, or with added neural structures – lipomyelomeningocele. A rare type of cystic SBO is terminal myelocystocele. Another SBO variant without cystic component are the most common type of SBO. They comprise diastematomyelia, diplomyelia, dermal sinus (with or without epidermoid or dermoid cyst), lipoma, teratoma and tethered spinal cord due to various causes (adhesion, thickened filum terminale w/o fat tissue.

Typically, they are not only covered with the skin, but also initially are not presented with any neurological symptoms at least in the new-born period. No other neuraxis defects are usually associated with them.

At the level of covered NTD, typically in the midline or near midline, usually some cutaneous stigmata, like hairy patch, dimple, naevus, skin pigment changes or even subcutaneous mass can be detected. Any skin defect along the spinous processes or paraspinal skin is suspicious from occult spinal dysraphism and need further investigation. Ultrasound can be useful for initial screening but cannot be used stand-alone. MRI is a definitive tool for diagnosis and evaluation of the defect.

If even clinical symptoms of occult spinal dysraphism presents, they are usually symptoms of tethered spinal cord manifested during growing up, when spinal cord is fixed at the same level as at birth and does not adapt to osseous spinal canal growth.

Problems usually start with voiding and stooling problems that can be overlooked in new-borns. Continuous drippling may attract attention and should prompt bladder volume measurement and urge urological and neurosurgical consulatations. Walking delay in children and contractures and deformities of lower extremities, back and legs pain, scoliosis, and onset of sphincter problems in childhood and adulthood justify the exclusion of OSD. Rarely recurrent neuroinfection can be the sign of OSD.

As usually no initial neurological deficit or other neuraxis malformation is present, question about indication for surgical repair arises. As many spina bifida occulta cases are diagnosed incidentally in adulthood, on graphical examination due to other problems, or even post-mortem, conservative management is a logical conclusion.

Against postponed surgery is fact, that surgery at the time of developed symptoms rarely reverse neurological deficit and intervention is successful if neurological deficit remains stable, with minimal possibility for improvement.

As sequalae of spina bifida occulta can be combination of symptoms including bladder dysfunction, orthopedic problems seriously limiting quality of life, preventive surgery or at least long-lasting meticulous patient's observation is recommended.

Cystic spina bifida occulta

As the surgery for SBO is indicated, there is no big difference with spina bifida aperta.

If meningocele covered with sufficient skin is indicated for surgery without signs of tethered spinal cord syndrome, e.g. for cosmetic reasons, after skin incision and identification and preparation of dural sac, just its resection and watertight dural suture without squeezing neural structure is the goal of surgery. Intradural inspection for any possible adhesions to spinal cord or thickened filum terminale is warranted. If there are clinical and radiographical signs of tethered spinal cord meticulous MRI evaluation must be done to rule out other sites of spinal cord fixation.

Lipomeningocele is another subtype of cystic SBO. The cyst is formed by dural protrusion filled with fat tissue which part of spinal cord within spinal canal. If the neural tissue is a part of the cyst, lesion is named as lipomyelomeningocele. Distinction of this two lesion is only didactic, because neural tissue is always an integral part of lesion and both are the results of the same pathology when premature disjunction of epithelial ectoderm from neural ectoderm occurs, allowing mesenchymal tissue come to contact with neural ectoderm, which stimulates mesenchyme to develop to fatty tissue. Ventrally is mesenchyme stimulated by neural plate to transform to meninges and interface between meninges and fat tissue is at neural ridge. Skin covering lesion is completely differentiated with possible skin marks. As the tethering of spinal cord is inherent to this lesion, surgery is indicated to prevent deterioration of preserved neural functions. If there is apparent soft tumor visible or palpable under the skin or if there are cutaneous stigmata suspicious from SBO or even suspicious tethered spinal cord syndrome based on clinical presentation HR MRI proves diagnosis (**Figure 8**) Urologic and urodynamic testing proves impairment of bladder function. Preoperative electrophysiological examination assesses lower sacral and coccygeal nerve roots functions. Electromyography of anal sphincter demonstrate 96% sensitivity of sphincter dyssynergia and 78% sensitivity in

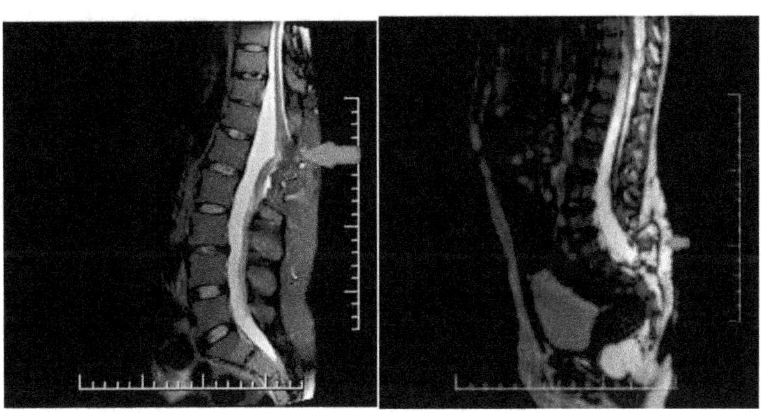

Figure 8.
Thoracic and lumbar lipomyelomeningocele (red arrows) on MRI.

bladder dysmotility detection. With perineal evoked potential added, sensitivity for sphincter dyssynergia increase to 100% and for bladder dysmotility to 86% [8].

Interface between neural placode and lipoma is indistinct. So, the aim of surgery is not to remove fat tissue intimately adherent to neural tissue, but deliberate spinal cord and reducing fatty mass, with preservation of neural structures, filum terminale resection and prevention of re-tethering. Lipoma may be resected using ultrasonic aspirator, cautery, even laser, while preserving neural structures intact. It is better left more fatty tissue on neural placode as do irreversible damage, while distinction between neural placode and lipoma is impossible even under microscopic control. For maximizing surgery safety, intraoperative electrophysiological monitoring using somatosensory evoked potential, motor evoked potential and electromyography including anal sphincter monitoring is necessary.

As the lipomyelomeningocele and lipomeningocele are of all spina bifida malformations most prone for retethering, generous duroplasty must be done to create copious space filled with CSF preventing postoperative adhesions. After watertight duroplasty, upper layers are closed in standard manner.

Postoperative complications and their management are like open spina bifida.

Terminal myelocystocele is a rarest form of cystic SBO, accounting about 4–8% of all OSD cases [9–11], which is defined as cystic dilatation of central canal protruding dorsally to subcutaneous tissue in lumbosacral region, usually coupled with another spinal, anorectal and genitourinal malformations. This malformation is caused by disruption of secondary neurulation resulting in persistent terminal vesicle and its expansion through dorsal mesenchyme but not epithelial ectoderm. Cystic dilatation is lined with ependymal cells and is continuous with central canal. Transition zone is funnel-like on MRI. At the basal site of the cyst is formed by placode, cranially continuous with spinal cord. Usually this malformation, besides subcutaneous mass and cutaneous stigmata is presented with neurological deficit, but cases without no neurological disturbance had been referred [9].

Spinal cord fixation is always associated with this lesion, so detethering is indicated. There is no imminent threat of neurological deterioration and surgery can be done electively. The principle of intervention is releasing spinal cord and placode and if possible, neural tube reconstruction. Starting with midline incision above lesion and resection of fat tissue/lipoma to identify dural sac. If necessary, cranial laminectomy allows better identification of dura. After dural opening cyst is in view, with possible adhesions. Any fixations also of spinal cord in operative field must be released. After cyst resection at the bottom placode is visible. After neural placode, spinal cord and nerve roots identification, any fixation points of neural structure responsible for persistent or newly developed fixation must be unloosed. Reconstruction of placode using 5/0 monofilament nonabsorbable pial sutures prevents retethering. Dural reconstruction is done in standard manner, bearing in mind not to compress or squeeze underlying neural structures. Flap from adjacent paravertebral muscles fortify dural suture and prevent CSF oozing. Subcutaneous tissue and skin are closed in standard way. After surgery prone position with slightly elevated hips helps wound healing. Due to surgical site localization nearby anus, infection prevention is particularly important.

In addition to the caudal end of spinal canal, myelocystocele can be found wherever along the spine. Neurological impairment is defined by the malformation level. Surgery is performed in the standard manner described above.

Spinal lipoma

Spinal lipomas are the most frequent varieties of non-cystic SBO. They are mature teratomas, consisting of mature adipocytes, which react to metabolic stimuli like fat tissue anywhere in the body, what may influence their clinical presentation.

The fillar lipoma, lipoma as a part of filum terminale, is the most common type of intradural lipoma. It is estimated incidence is about 1–5% and symptomatic are about 5% of them [12].

Filum terminale is infiltrated with fat in various extend. Commonly caudal nerve roots are not involved or compressed. If the filum terminale lipoma is symptomatic, it is usually associated with low lying conus medullaris and tethered cord syndrome. As asymptomatic cases are not usually diagnosed and diagnosis is made incidentally, there is not strict indication for surgery. On the other hand, filum terminale resection is surgery associated with low risk and can prevent later deterioration.

In symptomatic cases, surgery of filum terminale resection at the level of lipoma, through midline incision, laminectomy and durotomy is indicated.

Conus medullaris lipomas are distinct category of lipomas in lumbar spine, which are broadly adherent to lumbar spinal cord. Usually are associated with cystic spina bifida. As the fat tissue is intimately connected with neural tissue, complete resection is rarely possible. Intraoperative neuromonitoring is necessary for surgery safety.

Classical intradural lipomas occur along whole spinal canal, with predominant location in lumbosacral region. They are enclosed in normally formed dural sac. Their localization defines their clinical presentation, caused by spinal cord compression. As mentioned before, their separation from neural tissue is difficult, so partial resection with duroplasty is principle of surgery.

Split cord malformation

Split cord malformation (SCM) is category of OSD which includes two subtypes – diastematomyelia and diplomyelia. According generally accepted theory, these two types are variations from opposite sides of one developmental failure as proposed by Pang [13].

In diastematomyelia, type I., there are two hemicords, each with its own dural covering, separated by septum. Septum is composed of connective tissue, usually bone. Also, cartilaginous septum or spur can separate this hemicords. Septum is in general composed also of other types of connective tissue, including blood vessels. Arteries can be huge and making surgery difficult. Septum can be localized more laterally to either side or can be oblique in relation to spinal canal axis. This type is usually associated with vertebral anomalies.

In type II., diplomyelia, there are two cords enclosed in common dural sleeve, usually separated with fibrous septum, attached to ventral and dorsal dura. There are identified three types of septa according its attachment to dura. One type is only septum attached to the dorsal circumference, another with attachment to ventral dura and the last one traversing all internal diameter of dural sac. Septal attachment to the dura is usually localized more caudally as its attachment to the cleft between hemicords, as a sign of spinal cord tethering.

The embryologic basis of pathology is still in question.

Although some SCM are diagnosed prenatally, most of them are diagnosed after delivery or even in adulthood. At the birth neurological status is normal or almost normal. SCM is associated with cutaneous stigmata. CT and MRI are diagnostic tools capable to identify not only two hemicords, but also character of septum and identification vessels in it.

Clinical presentation is associated with spinal cord fixation, presenting with tethered cord syndrome, usually in type I., while the diplomyelia can be asymptomatic, but as a possible source of spinal cord tethering with insidious neurological deficit progression, when diagnosed, is also indication for surgical treatment.

In the type I. SCM (diastematomyelia), after midline skin incision above lesion and posterior bony structures are skeletonized, laminectomy above and below lesion is performed. It is sometimes tricky, because in this type of SCM laminae used to be hypertrophic and fused. After identification of dura at the sites of laminectomies, laminectomy on the top of lesion, from lateral to medial is done up to septum. Next step is removing intervening septum, what may be challenging step because of vessels in it. In this step bone wax or haemostatic material is helpful. Dura above and below split cord is opened, and unified spinal cord is identified. Dural opening continues above both hemicords. Medial adhesions between hemicords and dura are sharply cut. Some aberrant nerve roots, ending in medially located dura, can be identified, and interrupted. Medial dura is resected. There is no need to close ventral dura. Dorsal dura is closed in standard watertight manner, and if needed, with graft. Muscles, fascia, subcutaneous tissue, and skin is closed standardly.

The type ll. laminectomy is usually easier to do because laminae used to be more delicate. After exposure of dura, there are usually no signs of intradural septa visible from outside. Sometimes this pathology is associated with meningocele manque, which must be distinguished from septum. Paramedial vertical durotomy is done. After elevation of dorsal dura, posterior circumference of spinal cord is inspected. If there is septum, must be sharply bisected. Along the septum are sometimes vessels resembling arteriovenous malformation or aberrant nerve roots. If possible, vessel should be preserved. In this type of SCM both hemicords are in intime relation, so ventral inspection through the medial cleft is not recommended. Gentle rotation of spinal cord usually allows visualization of ventral dura and safe section of septum. Watertight dural closure and wound suture is done in standard manner.

Dermal sinus tract

Dermal sinus tract (DST) is a form of occult spinal dysraphism. Incidence of this malformation is estimated to 1 in 2500 live births [14].

This type of OSD is characterized by tract between skin and deeper structures. It is result of impaired disjunction between dermal and neural ectoderm at the 3rd to 8th gestation week. Majority of referred cases are in lumbar and sacral region. Epithelial-lined tract can end in variable depths ranging from subcutaneous tissue to dural sac, which is the most frequent its termination and used to be associated with intradural inclusion tumor, i.e. dermoid/epidermoid tumor, even teratoma. Cutaneous stigmata are associated with DST in 77.1%, what can help differentiate DST from benign sacrococcygeal pits [15].

In the case of transdural penetration DST is associated with tethered cord syndrome. Dermal sinus tract can be reason of repetitive neuroinfection. Source of infections is usually external, passing through the tract, but inflammation can also be caused by chemical irritation from leakage of dermoid cyst content.

Different incidence of clinical symptoms is referred in literature ranging from up to 1% [16] to 75% [14].

If there is clinical suspicion of DST, its probing is not recommended. Primary diagnostic tool is ultrasound with its specificity 98% [17].

Definitive diagnosis is confirmed by MRI, which can reveal not only tract, but also its relation to dural sac and any intradural pathology (**Figure 9**).

Although MRI does not identify tract traversing through dural sac, surgical treatment is indicated. Despite high sensitivity of MRI, narrow tract ending in dural sac can be unidentified on MRI.

Surgery is performed with midline skin with elliptical incision encircling external ostium. Tract is followed until its end is identified, even if unplanned laminectomy must be done. If there is a contact with dura mater, part of dura encircling tract is excised with intradural revision. Intradural pathology, if identified accidentally, or identified preoperatively, are dealt according its nature.

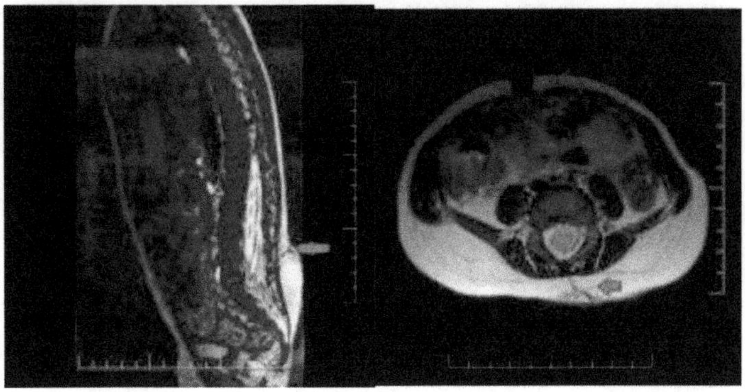

Figure 9.
Dermal sinus tract extending to the dura mater (red arrows) on sagittal and coronal MRI.

Dermoid/epidermoid, teratoma tumors are excised. Internal decompression of dermoid/epidermoid tumors increases the safety of the operation and aids in complete excision. Any part of the left tumor is a potential source of recurrence. Any adhesions to spinal cord must be released and filum terminal, if is accessible is indicated for resection. Wound closure is done in standard manner. Prone position after surgery is preferred.

Meningocele manqué

Special type of neural tube defect is so called meningocele manqué. In this type of malformation spinal cord, nerve roots or filum terminal are fixed by fibrous band formed by atrophic or incomplete meningoceles. These fibrous bands can pass through all soft back tissues ending at the skin or can end on lamina or be fixed to dura mater. This is like reverse dermal sinus tract.

Clinical presentation is identical to tethered spinal cord syndrome, consisting of reflex changes on lower extremities, progressive weakness, muscle dystonia, pain and/or bladder dysfunction.

Suspicion arises with cutaneous stigmata as described before.

Even with evident clinical presentation, there might no sign on MRI of spinal cord fixation with conus localized at the typical L1/L2 disc level. Thorough MRI scans examination, especially high resolution CISS MRI can be helpful in diagnostic hesitation.

If there is a proved, or suspect intradural spinal cord fixation correlating with clinical presentation, surgery, even exploratory, aimed to releasing any adhesions, is recommended. To minimize risk of perioperative neurological injury, perioperative monitoring is inevitable.

Surgery of accompanied pathologies

Hydrocephalus

Hydrocephalus is often, up to 85% of new-born with SB, associated disease. It may be identified prenatally on ultrasound or may be identified or develop after delivery. According to multiple observations, the higher is the spinal lesion localized, shunt dependent hydrocephalus is more probable [18].

Pathophysiology of hydrocephalus associated with spinal dysraphism is still in question. CSF leakage through spinal canal defect causes lowering CSF pressure intracranially resulting in circulation and resorption pathways non-development. After open spina bifida repair missing CSF resorption mechanism results in its accumulation and hydrocephalus.

Obstruction of CSF outflow due to hindbrain protrusion to the spinal canal may be the source of hydrocephalus development.

In the case of apparent hydrocephalus, MRI is indicated to exclude other reasons of obstruction of CSF pathways.

Timing of surgery is still in question. In the case of apparent hydrocephalus identified in utero or at birth, hydrocephalus surgery together with spina bifida aperta closure is recommended. One stage surgery of hydrocephalus and open spina bifida helps wound healing by reducing CSF pressure, reduce risk of CSF leakage and infection.

Doubts arise in the case of no clinical/graphical signs of postnatal hydrocephalus. Ventricular volume may be reduced because of CSF loss through open spinal defect. After defect closure, intraventricular CSF accumulation occurs and head circumference rises, but not necessarily due to pathologically elevated ICP and hydrocephalus. In new-borns calvarium bones are cartilaginous with open sutures, intracranial pressure reflects skin elasticity. Tendency is to avoid invasive procedures unless they are necessary, so MRI and CT are not useful in ventricular size monitoring because of radiation and/or need for anesthesia. Also, invasive ICP monitoring is not the solution. The best option for monitoring, except for direct biparietal, fronto-occipital and circumferential measurement on daily basis, ultrasound monitoring, also with Doppler sonography, is best practical option [19].

In surgery indication is necessary bear in mind that the young age and the small blood mass of the patients is not in favor of a long surgical intervention.

There are two main options for surgery. Ventriculoperitoneal shunt insertion is a standard hydrocephalus therapy, bearing higher risk of failure due to obstruction, infection, mechanical failure. As surgery is done on new-borns, up to adulthood, with exclusion shunt failure or infection, revision will be necessary at least due to patient's growth.

If ventriculoperitoneal drainage is indicated, ventricular catheter may be inserted into the frontal, occipital horn or trigonum in supposed non-dominant hemisphere. Site of insertion depends on surgeons' preferences. The shorter is extracranial segment of drainage, the smaller is probability of ventricular catheter dislocation outside ventricle with the head growth. Occipital horn insertion is associated with less probability of catheter obstruction by chorioid plexus with sufficient length of catheter placed intraventricularly. Frontal horn allows efficient portion of catheter to be inserted in ventricle with easy positioning for ventriculoperitoneal shunt, without need of patient repositioning during surgery. A little higher incidence of obstruction by chorioid plexus is associated with frontal horn drainage. Ventricular trigone allows shorter intraventricular length of catheter, but also shortest extracranial portion of ventricular catheter.

Ventriculoperitoneal shunt is completed in standard manner. Curvilinear incisions are preferred for exclusion contact points between parts of shunt system (catheters, valve, antisiphon unit) and edges of wound to minimize risk of infection and relieve pressure on the skin suture. In new-born non-toothed forceps for skin manipulation is preferred, and reduced coagulation prevents necrosis and wound healing problems including infection. Ventricular catheter insertion should be done after distal part is prepared for insertion. That means, valve with antisiphon unit are in retoauricular subcutaneous pocket connected with connected peritoneal catheter, which is tunneled to the paraumbilical incision, where intraperitoneal approach is prepared at least, up to dorsal fascia. After ventricular catheter is inserted and tunneled with shunt passer into the retoauricular pouch, then connected with valve and all connection are secured with silk tie. Before intraperitoneal insertion verification of functional system must be done. Both cranial wounds are closed in layers.

There are others, less used, insertions of distal catheter. It can be inserted into the venous system through tributaries of external jugular vein. In this approach, any shunt infection is associated with sepsis.

Prophylactic antibiotics are indicated.

In the case of contraindication of longer surgery, or any pathology, which prevents intraperitoneal insertion, external ventricular drainage is an option or subcutaneous reservoir (Omaya, Rickham).

Endoscopic third ventriculostomy, because of higher risk of failure before 6 months of age, is an option if revision due to previously inserted drainage is indicated [20].

Chiari ll. malformation

Chiari malformation type ll. is herniation of hindbrain into the cervical spinal canal and is exclusively associated with spina bifida.

While Chiari ll. malformation was not observed during embryonal development and is detectable during foetal stage of development, it is believed to be not primary malformation, but reflexes changed environment due to different CSF pressure gradients in case of open spina bifida [21, 22].

With lower pressure in CSF spaces intracranially, stimulation for posterior cranial fossa enlargement is reduced and posterior fossa neural tissue grows in standard manner. This theory is supported by MOMS study when in utero myelomeningocele closure significantly reduces Chiari ll. Malformation incidence [23].

Despite, it is usually asymptomatic (**Figure 10**), when symptomatic, its manifestation is life threatening. Clinical presentations, such as trunk and limbs muscle tonus impairment, dysphagia, stridor and vocal cord palsy, weak cry, central apnea manifest after delivery, during childhood and adulthood or never. According to present information, there is no correlation between presenting clinical symptoms and severity of anatomical severity compression on MRI.

Most accepted theory, why herniation occurs is disturbance of CSF pressure gradient between intracranial and spinal part of CSF compartment due to CSF leakage through neural tube defect.

Applying this theory in symptomatic Chiari malformation, type 2, the reasonable treatment is by lowering ICP.

As a primal type of surgery ventriculo-peritoneal shunt is usually applied in older children and adults.

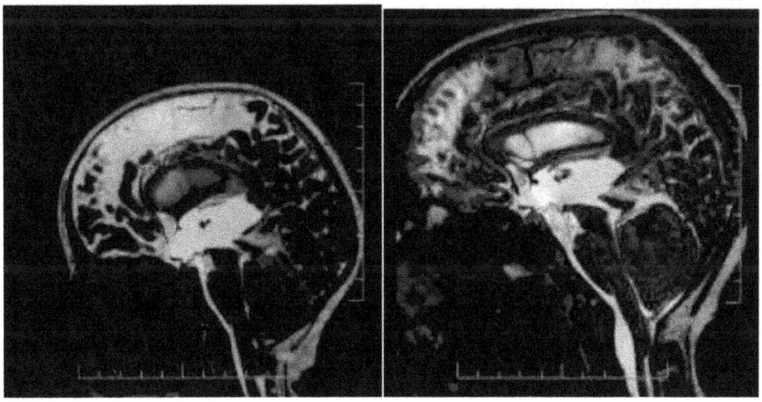

Figure 10.
Chiari ll. Malformation identified at the time of myelomeningococele closure on left picture (red arrow points to herniation) resolves completely four years after surgery – Right picture.

New-born and infants are usually treated primarily with external ventricular drainage with later internalization when effectiveness of ICP lowering on clinical symptoms improvement was proved.

In the cases of persisted clinical symptoms cervico-cranial decompression comes to role. Despite foramen magnum is enlarged, suboccipital craniectomy with preferred laminoplasty over laminectomy on upper cervical vertebrae relieve compression on neural structures. Extend of cervical decompression is planned according preoperative MRI. Torcular identification on MRI and bearing in mind its localization prevents massive intraoperative bleeding with possible menacing consequences, when dura is opened, despite there no consensus about necessity of duroplasty [24].

Because spinal and cranial dura lacks elasticity consisting mostly of collagen fibers duroplasty is recommended.

Because of distorted anatomy associated with high risk of neural or vascular damage, arachnoideal dissection to explore the fourth ventricle and normal spinal cord identification is reserved only for cases with syringomyelia [25].

Artificial dura is used to complete duroplasty with sufficient space for neural content and CSF. Dural sealants reduce CSF leakage. Wound is closed in layers.

Approximately one tenths of patients require reoperation. Reason for recurrent compression can be extensive epidural scaring or new bone formation.

3. Conclusions

The treatment of spina bifida is a complex problem that requires multidisciplinary treatment not only at the time of surgery, but also often requires lifelong medical follow-up and therapy.

Acknowledgements

This chapter is published with grant VEGA 1/0428/21 support.

Conflict of interest

Author has no conflict of interest.

Acronyms and Abbreviations

CSF	cerebrospinal fluid
ICP	intracranial pressure
VPS	ventriculoperitoneal shunt (VPS)
DST	dermal sinus tract (DST)
SCT	spinal cord tethering
SB	spina bifida
SBO	spina bifida occulta
SCM	split cord malformation
AFP	alpha fetoprotein (AFP)
OSD	occult spinal dysraphism

Author details

Juraj Šutovský
Jessenius Faculty of Medicine in Martin, University Hospital Martin,
Comenius University in Bratislava, Martin, Slovakia

*Address all correspondence to: jsutovsky@unm.sk

References

[1] Williams J, Mai CT, Mulinare J, Isenburg J, Flood TJ, Ethen M, et al. Centers for Disease Control and Prevention. Updated estimates of neural tube defects prevented by mandatory folic acid fortification - United States, 1995-2011. MMWR. Morbidity and Mortality Weekly Report. 2015 Jan 16;**64**(1):1-5 25590678; PMCID: PMC4584791

[2] Schulz LN, Tecle NE, Cleary R, Mercier P. Spontaneous closure of myelomeningocele. Child's Nervous System. 2020 Apr;**36**(4):869-871. DOI: 10.1007/s00381-019-04454-z. Epub 2020 Feb 5 32025870

[3] Boyd PA, Haeusler M, Barisic I, Loane M, Garne E, Dolk H. Paper 1: The EUROCAT network--organization and processes. Birth Defects Research. Part A, Clinical and Molecular Teratology. 2011 Mar;**91**(Suppl 1):S2-S15. DOI: 10.1002/bdra.20780. Epub 2011 Mar 7 21384531

[4] Pang D. Surgical complications of open spinal dysraphism. Neurosurgery Clinics of North America 1995 Apr;6(2):243-257. PMID: 7620351.

[5] Yun-Hai S, Nan B, Ping-Ping G, Bo Y, Cheng C. Is repair of the protruded meninges sufficient for treatment of meningocele? Childs Nerv Syst. 2015 Nov;31(11):2135-40. doi: 10.1007/s00381-015-2874-4. Epub 2015 Aug 23. PMID: 26298824; PMCID: PMC4617846.

[6] Moldenhauer JS, Adzick NS. Fetal surgery for myelomeningocele: After the Management of Myelomeningocele Study (MOMS). Seminars in Fetal & Neonatal Medicine. 2017 Dec;**22**(6):360-366. DOI: 10.1016/j.siny.2017.08.004. Epub 2017 Oct 12 29031539

[7] Mazzola CA, Tyagi R, Assassi N, Bauer DF, Beier AD, Blount JP, et al. Congress of Neurological Surgeons systematic review and evidence-based guideline on the incidence of tethered cord syndrome in infants with myelomeningocele with prenatal versus postnatal repair. Neurosurgery. 2019 Sep 1;**85**(3):E417-E419. DOI: 10.1093/neuros/nyz266 31418037

[8] Torre M, Planche D, Louis-Borrione C, Sabiani F, Lena G, Guys JM. Value of electrophysiological assessment after surgical treatment of spinal dysraphism. The Journal of Urology. 2002 Oct;**168**(4 Pt 2):1759-1762; discussion 1763. DOI: 10.1097/01.ju.0000030855.05366.6d 12352354

[9] Kumar R, Chandra A. Terminal myelocystocele. Indian Journal of Pediatrics. 2002 Dec;**69**(12):1083-1086. DOI: 10.1007/BF02724394 12557964

[10] McLone DG, Naidich TP. Terminal myelocystocele. Neurosurgery 1985 Jan;16(1):36-43. PMID: 3883218.

[11] Mirza B, Mahmood N, Ijaz L, Khawaja T, Aslam I, Sheikh A. Isolated terminal myelocystocele: A rare spinal dysraphism. APSP J Case Rep. 2011 Jan;**2**(1):3. Epub 2011 Mar 10. PMID: 22953270 PMC3418015

[12] Cools MJ, Al-Holou WN, Stetler WR Jr, Wilson TJ, Muraszko KM, Ibrahim M, La Marca F, Garton HJ, Maher CO. Filum terminale lipomas: Imaging prevalence, natural history, and conus position. Journal of Neurosurgery. Pediatrics 2014 May;13(5):559-567. doi: 10.3171/2014.2.PEDS13528. Epub 2014 Mar 14. PMID: 24628511.

[13] Pang D, Dias MS, Ahab-Barmada M. Split cord malformation: Part I: A unified theory of embryogenesis for double spinal cord malformations. Neurosurgery. 1992 Sep;**31**(3):451-480. DOI: 10.1227/00006123-199209000-00010 1407428

[14] Ackerman LL, Menezes AH. Spinal congenital dermal sinuses: A 30-year experience. Pediatrics. 2003 Sep;**112**(3 Pt 1):641-647. DOI: 10.1542/peds.112.3.641 12949296

[15] Radmanesh F, Nejat F, El Khashab M. Dermal sinus tract of the spine. Child's Nervous System 2010 Mar;26(3):349-357. doi: 10.1007/s00381-009-0962-z. Epub 2009 Aug 7. PMID: 19662426.

[16] Pang D. Split cord malformation: Part II: Clinical syndrome. Neurosurgery. 1992 Sep;**31**(3):481-500. DOI: 10.1227/00006123-199209000-00011 1407429

[17] Chern JJ, Aksut B, Kirkman JL, Shoja MM, Tubbs RS, Royal SA, et al. The accuracy of abnormal lumbar sonography findings in detecting occult spinal dysraphism: A comparison with magnetic resonance imaging. Journal of Neurosurgery. Pediatrics. 2012 Aug;**10**(2):150-153. DOI: 10.3171/2012.5.PEDS11564. Epub 2012 Jun 29 22747088

[18] Rintoul NE, Sutton LN, Hubbard AM, Cohen B, Melchionni J, Pasquariello PS, et al. A new look at myelomeningoceles: Functional level, vertebral level, shunting, and the implications for fetal intervention. Pediatrics. 2002 Mar;**109**(3):409-413. DOI: 10.1542/peds.109.3.409 11875133

[19] Kolarovszki B, Zubor P, Kolarovszka H, Benco M, Richterova R, Matasova K. The assessment of intracranial dynamics by transcranial doppler sonography in perioperative period in paediatric hydrocephalus. Archives of Gynecology and Obstetrics. 2013 Feb;**287**(2):229-238. DOI: 10.1007/s00404-012-2576-z. Epub 2012 Sep 25 23008112

[20] Vulcu S, Eickele L, Cinalli G, Wagner W, Oertel J. Long-term results of endoscopic third ventriculostomy: An outcome analysis. Journal of Neurosurgery. 2015 Dec;**123**(6):1456-1462. DOI: 10.3171/2014.11.JNS14414. Epub 2015 Jul 31 26230473

[21] McLone DG, Knepper PA. The cause of Chiari II malformation: A unified theory. Pediatric Neuroscience. 1989;**15**(1):1-12. DOI: 10.1159/000120432 2699756

[22] Osaka K, Tanimura T, Hirayama A, Matsumoto S. Myelomeningocele before birth. Journal of Neurosurgery. 1978 Nov;**49**(5):711-724. DOI: 10.3171/jns.1978.49.5.0711 712393

[23] Farmer DL, Thom EA, Brock JW 3rd, Burrows PK, Johnson MP, Howell LJ, Farrell JA, Gupta N, Adzick NS; Management of Myelomeningocele Study Investigators. The Management of Myelomeningocele Study: full cohort 30-month pediatric outcomes. Am J Obstet Gynecol. 2018 Feb;218(2):256.e1-256.e13. doi: 10.1016/j.ajog.2017.12.001. Epub 2017 Dec 12. PMID: 29246577.

[24] Alford EN, Hopson BD, Safyanov F, Arynchyna A, Bollo RJ, Hankinson TC, et al. Care management and contemporary challenges in spina bifida: A practice preference survey of the American Society of Pediatric Neurosurgeons. Journal of Neurosurgery. Pediatrics. 2019 Aug;**30**:1-10. DOI: 10.3171/2019.5.PEDS18738. Epub ahead of print 31470398

[25] Talamonti G, Marcati E, Mastino L, Meccariello G, Picano M, D'Aliberti G. Surgical management of Chiari malformation type II. Child's Nervous System. 2020 Aug;**36**(8):1621-1634. DOI: 10.1007/s00381-020-04675-7. Epub 2020 May 30 32474814

Chapter 4

Urologic Implications and Management in Spina Bifida

Adrián Gutiérrez-González, José Iván Robles-Torres and Daniel García-Sánchez

Abstract

Urological disorders, including urinary infections, incontinence, and renal failure, represent a significant source of morbidity and mortality in these patients. Long-term mortality is associated to urological causes in approximately 33%. In order to prevent this complications, urologic evaluation since early childhood must be done. The evaluation of the degree of damage to the urinary tract and the determination of the type of neurogenic bladder involved in the spina bifida spectrum will be the guideline for establishing therapeutic management, which can be from behavioral modifications, medical management, minimally invasive therapy and, as a last resort, surgery. In this chapter, we will discuss the wide spectrum of urologic implications, a brief reminder of urinary tract physiology and the pathological processes involved in spina bífida, as well as long-term complications. The diagnostic evaluation of urinary tract and the different therapeutic modalities according to the type of neurogenic bladder and age will be discussed.

Keywords: urology, urinary tract infections, chronic kidney failure, management, augmentation cystoplasty, intermittent bladder catheterization

1. Introduction

1.1 The bladder and manifestations associated with spina bifida

The abnormal development of the neural tube is considered the most common cause of neurogenic bladder dysfunction in children. Nearly all patients with myelomeningocele (over 90%) will have some type of bladder dysfunction (neurogenic bladder), and 30–40% of these children will develop some degree of renal disease as a long-term complication if treatment is not implemented at an early age in childhood. [1]

Depending on the severity of the fusion defect and its location, a variety of neurological deficits can be seen, with variable impact on somatic, parasympathetic and sympathetic innervation of the bladder. For unclear reasons, the level of the lesion correlates poorly with urodynamics findings and the severity of lower urinary tract dysfunction. [2] This affects its ability to store and empty urine and can lead to chronic kidney disease by poor bladder dynamics. Urological problems, including urinary tract infections, incontinence, and renal failure, are a significant cause of morbidity and mortality. Long term mortality is associated to urological complications in approximately 33% of these patients. [3]

Children with myelomeningocele also have increased risk of developing kidney stones. In one study, the prevalence of kidney stones was 4 percent among children with spinal dysraphism, compared with 0.2 percent in healthy children. Likely mechanisms for this predisposition to upper tract urolithiasis include immobility (with resultant bone resorption), bacteriuria, and urinary stasis. [4]

The bladder is a hollow muscular organ whose function is to store urine to about 400–500 mL in adults and to void as a consequence of a consequence of a filling stimulus. The micturition cycle is the continuous event of storing and voiding of urine. Normal micturition lasts approximately 15–20 seconds, and typically the bladder empties seven times a day and, usually, never at night. Under normal conditions, the bladder works at low pressures constantly. That means that during filling phase, its pressure does not exceed 10 cmH20. This condition allows the continuous gravitational flow of urine from the ureter to the bladder, and not vice versa. When, for abnormal conditions, the pressure in the bladder exceeds 40 cmH20, urine flow stops and flows back to the ureters, causing their dilatation, and in the long term alteration of kidney function, culminating in end-stage chronic kidney disease if not treated promptly. Chronic kidney disease is one of the most frequent causes of mortality in patients with spina bifida. [5]

After surgical management, walking with or without aids can be achieved in all patients with sacral levels and 95% with low lumbar lesions, while lower urinary tract (LUT) dysfunction tends to remain as large post-void residual volume, high voiding pressures, and urinary incontinence. In contrast, in patients with occult spina bifida, most cases are incidentally found during X-ray screening of low back pain. The vast majority is asymptomatic. Some cases are accompanied by lipomeningomyelocele, dermoid cyst, or thick flum terminale with minimum skin changes such as a dimple and focal hypertrichosis. In this scenario, LUT dysfunction may present in late childhood or in adulthood, and the severity of symptoms can vary, from nocturnal enuresis to urinary retention. In other words, the impact of the LUT will depend on the type of spinal dysraphism, whether it is a cystic or it is limited to an occult presentation.

The pattern of dysfunction caused by spinal dysraphism is determined by the site and type of lesion. Patterns are divided in three regions: the region above the pons, the region between the pons and the sacral cord, and the sacral cord and infrasacral region. Each region has particularities in bladder function. It is important to clarify that the manifestations according to this classification are not exact in all cases. The presentation of the neurogenic bladder in spina bifida is unpredictable. The clinical manifestations tend to present great heterogeneity. These mixed lesions can occur especially with lesions in close proximity of the conus medullaris. [6]

A detailed description of the most frequent sites affected by spina bifida are explained below:

1.2 Infrapontine-suprasacral lesions

A spinal cord lesion above the lumbosacral level, depending on completeness of the lesion, may eliminate (complete lesions) or at least reduce (incomplete lesions) voluntary cerebral control of micturition leading to neurogenic detrusor overactivity mediated by spinal reflex pathways. Detrusor overactivity has important clinical implications: reduced bladder capacity, detrusor-sphincter dyssynergia with post-void residual urine, incontinence, and a high intravesical pressure, which translates to a higher risk for chronic kidney disease. Severity of the clinical

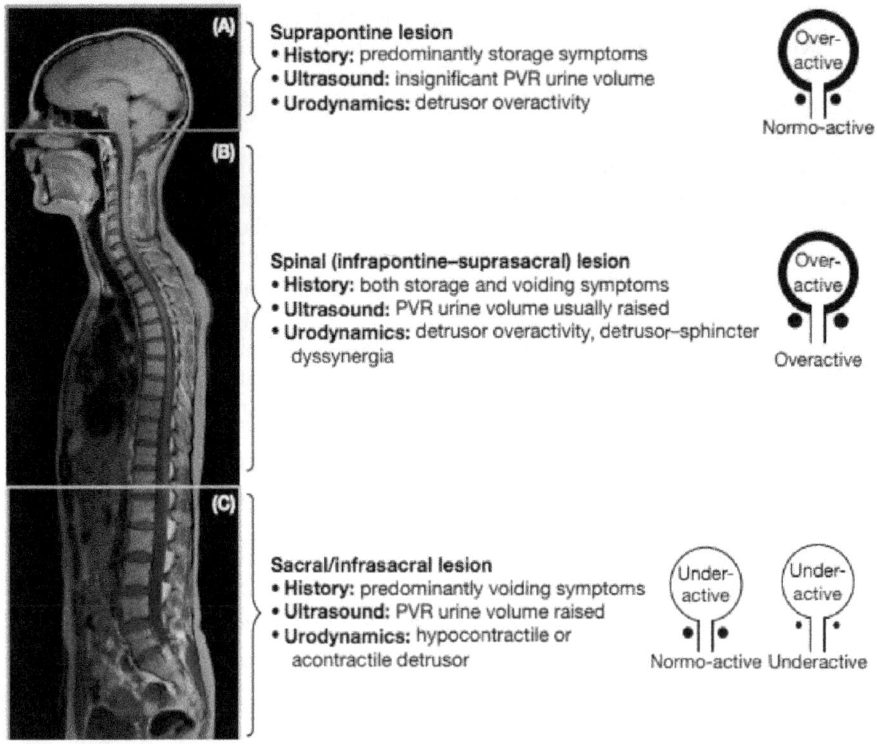

Figure 1.
Patterns of bladder dysfunction caused by neurological disorders: (A) Suprapontine lesion pattern; (B) Infrapontine-suprasacral pattern; (C) Sacral/infrasacral lesion pattern.

manifestations will depend on a complete injury is present and the level of injury (the higher, the more aggressive).

1.3 Sacral-infrasacral lesions

Lesions in this site will have predominantly voiding symptoms related to a hypocontractile (if incomplete lesion is present) or acontractile detrusor (complete lesion). The clinical presentation is due to injury to the parasympathetic motor nuclei that innervates the detrusor muscle. Stress urinary incontinence is usually related to Onuf's nucleus injury and pudendal nerve dysfunction over the striated sphincter (**Figure 1**).

2. Management of bladder storage and voiding symptoms

Lower urinary tract manifestations are divided into two groups: storage and voiding symptoms. Storage symptoms appear as an alteration in the filling phase of the micturition cycle. These symptoms include: increased voiding frequency, urgency, nocturia, urinary incontinence, and painful bladder syndrome.

Voiding symptoms appear as a difficulty during urination or prior to the onset of it. They include: difficulty to initiate urination, need to strain or effort to initiate and maintain urination, weak or intermittent urinary stream, terminal drip, dysuria and urgency. These symptoms result in incomplete voiding.

The primary goal of treatment is to preserve upper urinary tract function, improve continence, and improve quality of life in these patients. [5]

2.1 Storage management

In the scenario of the neurogenic patient associated with spinal dysraphism, the main complaint reported by patients is urinary incontinence, accompanied or not by urinary infections. Urinary incontinence can be explained by several pathophysiological mechanisms. Urodynamics is a useful tool that provides objective diagnostic information that allows us to know the specific cause of incontinence.

Treatment includes behavioral measures such as control of fluid intake and personal hygiene. The use of medications should always be combined with conservative measures. The aim of these drugs is to increase bladder capacity and decrease detrusor pressure. Anticholinergics (also named antimuscarinics) are the most commonly used drugs. Its efficacy has been demonstrated in neurogenic patients with urge urinary incontinence associated with an overactive detrusor. Beta 3 agonists are another option that was recently introduced. The efficacy of these drugs appears to be similar to anticholinergics with a non-inferior safety profile. The response to these medications is evaluated with the clinical control of incontinence, as well as an improvement in bladder capacity objectively observed by a decrease in detrusor pressure of less than 40 cmH2O when having a maximum bladder capacity in urodynamics. [5, 6]

2.2 Voiding symptoms

These patients are at a higher risk of presenting high filling pressures, which generates vesicoureteral reflux, resulting in dilatation of the upper urinary tract and deterioration of renal function. Chronic retention and reflux to the upper tract are conditions that increase the risk of urinary infections. Management focuses on improving and maintaining detrusor pressure below 40 cmH2O and control of urinary incontinence.

The use of clean intermittent catheterization as a mechanism for bladder emptying is considered the treatment of choice in the vast majority of neurogenic patients with evidence of urine retention. This treatment aims to adequately empty the bladder and thereby reduce urinary infections and incontinence. The use of an indwelling transurethral or suprapubic catheter should be avoided due to the demonstrated risks of recurrent urinary tract infections, stone formation, and urethral trauma [6] (**Figure 2**).

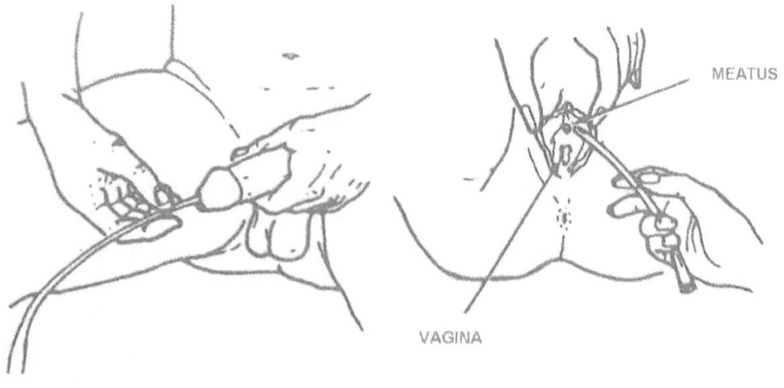

Figure 2.
Clean intermittent catheterization technique in male and female.

In patients where a functional voiding alteration is confirmed with dysfunction of the relaxation of the sphincter in the emptying phase of the micturition cycle, they can benefit from physiotherapy and biofeedback, which consist of training to improve bladder-sphincter coordination during urination. [5]

3. Follow-up protocol according to age

The main priority at the moment of birth is the closure of the spinal defect, as neurological complications are the main cause of morbidity and mortality during the first year of life; followed by urological complications. Specialized treatment centers state that the urological management should start immediately with intermittent catheterizations and anticholinergic medications due to the risk of collagen deposition in the bladder wall and consequent increased risk of upper urinary tract damage. In fact, each of the steps toward the management of this congenital disease are complex and the decisions may vary. [7]

3.1 Management from the moment of birth to the age of two years

A sonographic evaluation of the upper urinary tract as well as urine cultures are performed every 3 to 4 months. If both tests are normal, we wait until the age of 2 years, the age expected for most children to achieve voluntary control of micturition. In case of abnormal findings during any of the sonographic evaluations or 3 or more positive cultures accompanied with symptomatic infections during a year or less are encountered, it would be necessary to perform urodynamic testing complemented with a cystogram to discard any possibility of upper urinary tract damage due to a hostile bladder. If this is the case, it is time to start the adequate anticholinergic treatment and intermittent catheterizations. [8]

If no abnormal findings during this first 2-year follow-up are seen, an expectant management may be allowed.

3.2 Management from the age of two years to 20 years

Expectant management is modified to active management. Treatment goals are as follows: a) Avoidance of renal damage, b) Preservation of continence and c) Treatment of symptomatic urinary infections.

The first step is the functional evaluation by urodynamics and a structural evaluation with a cystogram. Videourodynamics is the Gold Standard as they are capable of evaluating both parameters. [9] A family member should be trained to perform clean intermittent catheterizations, so when the patient reaches the age of 6 years, this information should be passed onto the child to start self-intermittent catheterizations. We conducted a clinical trial in which we observed that intermittent catheterizations with clean technique using re-sterilized catheters did not increase neither the risk of urinary tract infection, nor bladder bacterial colonization. [10]

By performing urodynamic tests, the type of functional disturbance of the bladder may be assessed and classified in 4 types according to the Madersbacher classification: [11].

Type 1: High bladder pressure. High sphincter pressure.
Type 2: High bladder pressure. Low sphincter pressure.
Type 3: Low bladder pressure. High sphincter pressure.
Type 4: Low bladder pressure. Low sphincter pressure.

The risk of upper urinary tract damage is higher when Madersbacher type 1 and type 3 bladders are encountered. After identification of the bladder type, anticholinergic treatment should be started to normalize increased pressures. Three months after beginning of treatment, follow-up with a new urodynamic test is performed to assess the improvement of urodynamic parameters and clinical status.

The morphology of the bladder and the presence of vesicoureteral reflux (VUR) are assessed with a cystogram. The risk of vesicoureteral reflux in patients with neurogenic bladder is up to 17%. When VUR is observed, it is important to measure the detrusor pressure; if a pressure greater than 40 cmH20 is found, before thinking of any surgical treatment such as ureteral reimplantation, an attempt is made to decrease these pressures with conservative treatment. In case of success, a new evaluation is made to reassess if RUV disappeared (**Figure 3**) [12].

After functional and structural evaluation, proper bladder classification and having started initial treatment, the second stage of management is continued. Follow-up is made with urine cultures every 3 months, renal sonography every 6 months and renography every 1 to 3 years. Regarding the urodynamic test, when the detrusor pressure is greater than 40 cmH2O, the medical treatment is modified and a new urodynamic test is performed 3 months after, this is done until the goal of detrusor pressure of less than 40 cmH2O is achieved [13].

When to perform a new urodynamic test? 1) When there is less than 90% of voluntary micturition control. 2) When a new morphologic or functional disturbance of the kidney is observed. 3) Five years after the last urodynamic study. During this time, the type of neurogenic bladder could be modified due to the morphologic changes of growth and its effect on spinal cord. [14]

3.3 Management from the age of 21 years and over

When entering this stage, the patient is more aware of the disease and is more organized in its management. The bladder type usually reaches a stable state, and it is uncommon for the neurogenic bladder type to change. If this happens, it is important to evaluate the possibility of having a neurological disturbance that could need primary treatment.

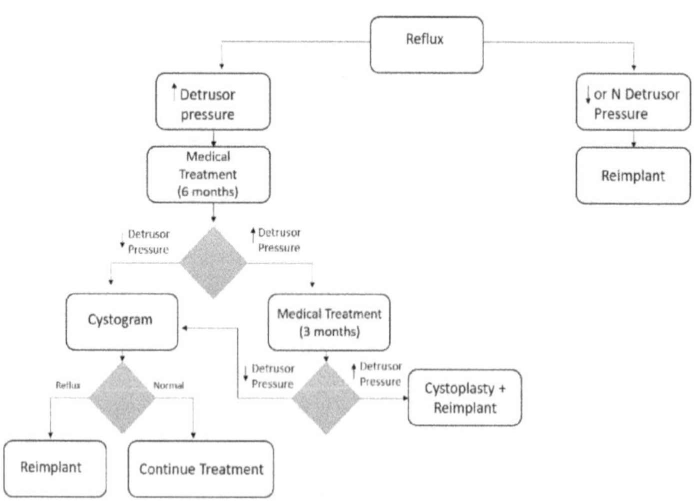

Figure 3.
Diagnostic and therapeutic algorithm in neurogenic bladder with vesico-ureteral reflux.

By this age, intermittent catheterizations are usually mastered by the patient and clinical signs that could be suspicious of active infection are well identified. Other topics, such as sexuality and reproduction are approached. Reproduction methods are informed and instructed; recommendations are given to women who wish to reproduce, such as folic acid intake and modifications on the route of administration of oxybutynin, from the oral to the intravesical route. [15]

On November 23rd of 1993, we founded the Spina Bifida Association in Moterrey, Mexico, where we presently have 1055 patients enrolled with the following age ranges:

< 15 years: 311 (29.5%)
16–29 years: 572 (54.2%)
>30 years 172 (16.3%)
Total: 1055 (100%)

A total of 472 (44.7%) patients assist with relative frequency (At least 3 consultations per year). Our experience has been forged working with the everyday management of our patients during 26 years, assessing their progression and deciding which procedures are the most adequate for them.

4. Urinary tract infections, when to treat?

Patients with neurogenic bladder due to spinal dysraphism have several factors that potentially increase the risk of urinary tract infections, such as, vesico-ureteral reflux (any grade), hypertonic bladder and foreign bodies inside the bladder. Schlager et al. observed that 70% of patients that perform intermittent bladder catheterizations present asymptomatic bacteriuria 24 weeks after the beginning of treatment. [16]

In patients with neurogenic bladder, including those secondary to myelomeningocele, urinary tract infections should be considered differently from those without any neurofunctional disease. The presence of bacteriuria within this group of patients is very common and unnecessary antibiotic treatment could be given if there is no acknowledgment of these facts. This could lead to future complications that develop due to antibiotic resistance and antibiotic side effects.

In patients performing intermittent bladder catheterizations, urine culture results with more than 10,000 CFU/ml are considered a clinical infection only when one or more of the following clinical features are present: foul smell, cloudy urine, fever of 38°C or more and abdominal or flank pain. [17] Positive urine culture without other clinical features is considered as bacterial colonization and requires no antibiotic treatment.

When deciding which antibiotic to prescribe, it is important to consider which antibiotics show the highest resistance within a community, which option would be delivered at adequate concentrations to the urinary bladder, this depending on the kidney's capacity to eliminate the active drug, and which would be more suitable to eliminate infection. It is important to ponder these considerations before antibiotic administration, as damage to the renal parenchyma may develop in a kidney already vulnerable to damage. [18]

Among the behavioral methods that help us in the prevention of urinary tract infections we include: Adequate liquid intake, maintenance of low postvoid urine and short time periods between intermittent catheterizations.

Intermittent bladder catheterization is a risk factor that predisposes to infection. There is no significant difference in the prevention of urinary tract infections when comparing the sterile technique with the clean technique, as well as with the use of a sterile catheter compared to a reused clean catheter; furthermore, the risk of colonization is the same between both techniques. [19]

5. Refractory cases to medical management

The objective of neurogenic bladder management secondary to myelomeningocele is focused on three main objectives: 1) Decrease the risk of renal damage 2) Preserve urinary continence and 3) Prevent urinary infection episodes. When these objectives are not reached with medical management, it is necessary to take more drastic decisions, otherwise, further problems regarding renal function may be encountered and quality of life may be affected. Such procedures include:

5.1 Neuromodulation

An attempt is made to modulate the nerve reflexes that control the bladder, sphincter and the pelvic floor through sacral nerve stimulation. The use of this technique is well documented in certain neurologically affected patients; however, in patients with myelomeningocele, there are controversial results due to structural abnormalities found at a sacral level, which makes this technique a lot harder. Evidence is still limited; however, this remains a continuous field of investigation (**Figure 4**) [20].

5.2 Augmentation cystoplasty

The aim of this procedure is to increase the bladder capacity and decrease elevated pressures in the urinary tract through an intestinal patch surgically fixed at the bladder dome. Some contraindications for these procedures are: 1) Any functional or structural disturbance of the gut, 2) Disturbances of hand dexterity to perform intermittent catheterizations, 3) Cognitive disturbances and 4) Significant damage to the renal function. [21] Significant changes have been observed after surgery regarding bladder storage as well as a decrease in filling pressure. Some early complications reported in the recent literature are wound infection (4–6%)

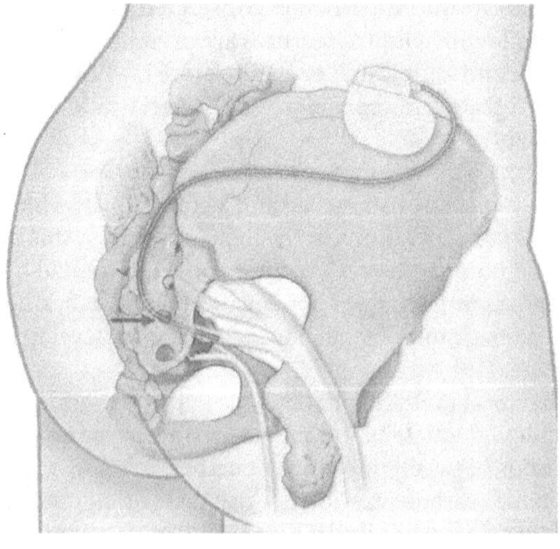

Figure 4.
Sacral neuromodulation therapy for refractory cases.

and intestinal obstruction (3–6%). The mortality rate within this group of patients is reported between 0 and 2.7%. Long-term complications include metabolic disturbances, such as hyperchloremia (16%) and decrease in renal function in patients with a creatinine clearance lower than 15 ml/min (15%) or higher than 40 ml/min (4.1%). [22] Mucus production by the intestinal lining is estimated between 35 and 40 gr/day, which predisposes to stone formation, infection and obstruction. After catheterizations, we perform intravesical irrigations with sodium bicarbonate at a dilution of 0.75% to reduce mucus thickness and attempt to reduce its production (**Figures 5–7**).

Perforation after bladder-gut anastomosis has been reported in 0.8–13% of procedures, occurring approximately 2 years after surgery, with a mortality rate of 25%. Risk of bladder cancer has been reported 10–20 years after surgery, and is believed to be caused by urinary stasis, nitrosamines, bladder stones, chronic inflammation of the intestinal patch and possible immune mechanisms with an estimated incidence of 10–20%. [23, 24]

Cystoscopy surveillance is recommended after a period of 10 years of surgery and in patients that develop hematuria, suprapubic pain or recurrent urinary tract infections.

5.3 Urinary diversion

Ileovesicostomy uses ileum as a bypass between the bladder and skin. This technique represents many clinical problems due to obstruction; furthermore, it predisposes to infections and bladder stones The Ileal conduit technique uses an

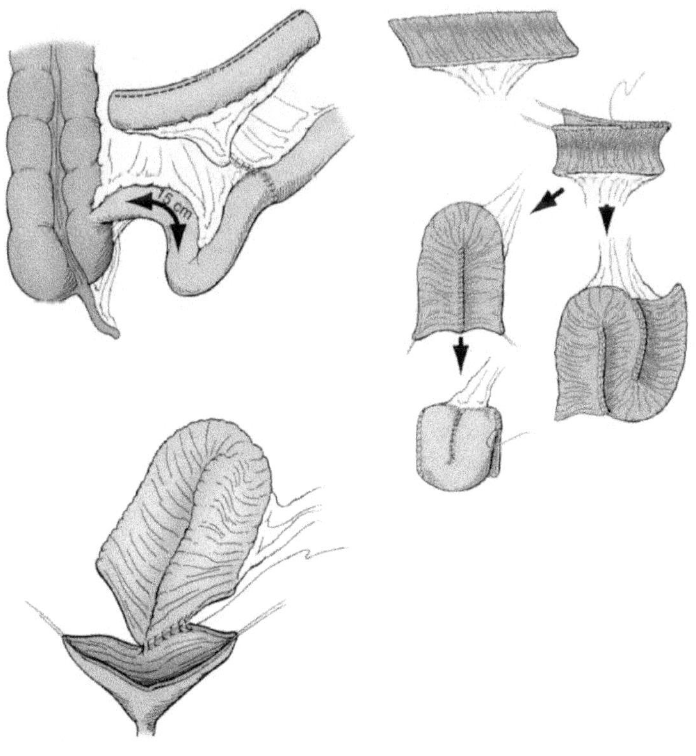

Figure 5.
Ileocistoplasty: a segment of ileum is remodeled and anastomosed to the bladder dome to increase the capacity of the bladder.

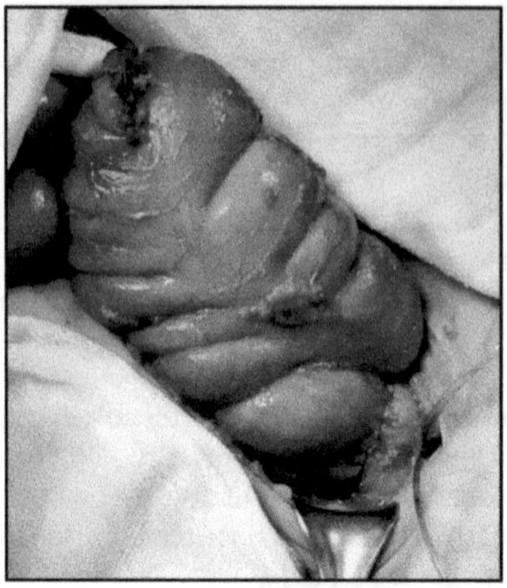

Figure 6.
Colocystoplasty: a segment of colon is remodeled and amastomosed to the bladder dome. Image obtain from hospital Universitario "Dr. José Eleuterio González", shared by Dr. Adrián Gutiérrez González.

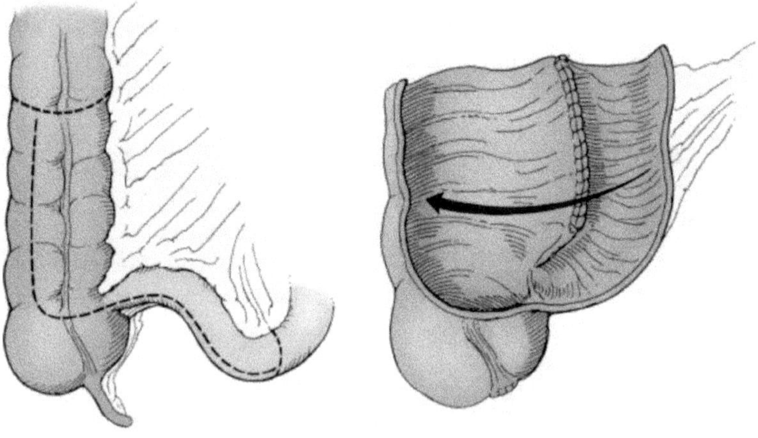

Figure 7.
Ileocecocystoplasty: Distal ileum and cecum are used to anastomose to the dome of the bladder.

ileum fragment which is closed at one end, both ureters are anastomosed to the conduit and the remaining open ileum end is connected to the abdominal wall, urine is collected by an external pouch. [25]

5.4 Catheter drainage

The permanent use of urinary catheters is not a good option due to the multiple complications that could develop. These include recurrent infections, meatal erosion, traumatic hypospadias, and stone formation. However, this technique can be used in cases with no other alternative options. If this were the case, the possibility of a suprapubic tube would be the most suitable option, which presents fewer complications. It is reserved only for patients with bladder emptying disturbances. This procedure is not recommended for patients with hyperactive neurogenic bladder, as urine leak surrounding the catheter entrance could appear. [26]

Author details

Adrián Gutiérrez-González[1,2*], José Iván Robles-Torres[1,2]
and Daniel García-Sánchez[1,2]

1 Hospital Universitario "Dr. José Eleuterio González", Universidad Autonoma de Nuevo León, Monterrey, Mexico

2 UroContinent, Monterrey, Mexico

*Address all correspondence to: dradriangtz@gmail.com

References

[1] Müller T, Arbeiter K, Aufricht C. Renal function in meningomyelocele: risk factors, chronic renal failure, renal replacement therapy and transplantation. Current opinion in urology. 2002 Nov 1;12(6): 479-84.

[2] Churchill BM, Abramson RP, Wahl EF. Dysfunction of the lower urinary and distal gastrointestinal tracts in pediatric patients with known spinal cord problems. Pediatr Clin North Am 2001;48(6):1587-630

[3] Snow-Lisy DC, Yerkes EB and Cheng EY: Update on urological management of spina bifida from prenatal diagnosis to adulthood. J Urol 2015;194: 288.

[4] Ramachandra P, Palazzi KL, Holmes NM, Chiang G. Children with spinal abnormalities have an increased health burden from upper tract urolithiasis. Urology. 2014 Jun 1;83(6):1378-82.

[5] Vignoli, G. *Urodynamics: A quick pocket guide*. Switzerland: Springer. 2017

[6] Dmochowski, R. R., & Heesakkers, J. *Neuro-Urology*. Cham: Springer. 2018

[7] Kaplan WE. Early evaluation and treatment of children with meningomyelocele. Problems in Urology. 1990 Jan 1;4(4):676-89.

[8] Mourtzinos A, Stoffel JT. Management goals for the spina bifida neurogenic bladder: a review from infancy to adulthood. Urologic Clinics. 2010 Nov 1;37(4):527-35.

[9] Marks BK, Goldman HB. Videourodynamics: indications and technique. The Urologic clinics of North America. 2014 Aug;41(3):383-9.

[10] Madero-Morales PA, Robles-Torres JI, Vizcarra-Mata G, Guillén-Lozoya AH, Mendoza-Olazarán S, Garza-González E, Gutiérrez-González A. Randomized clinical trial using sterile single use and reused polyvinylchloride catheters for intermittent catheterization with a clean technique in spina bifida cases: short-term urinary tract infection outcomes. The Journal of urology. 2019;202(1):153-8.

[11] Madersbacher H. The various types of neurogenic bladder dysfunction: an update of current therapeutic concepts. Spinal Cord. 1990 May;28(4):217-29.

[12] Snodgrass W, Villaneuva C, Jacobs M, Gargollo P. Upper tract changes in patients with neurogenic bladder and sustained pressures> 40 cm following bladder neck surgery without augmentation. Journal of pediatric urology. 2014 Aug 1;10(4):744-8.

[13] McGuire EJ, Woodside JR, Borden TA, Weiss RM. Prognostic value of urodynamic testing in myelodysplastic patients. The Journal of urology. 1981 Aug;126(2):205-9.

[14] Lew SM, Kothbauer KF. Tethered cord syndrome: an updated review. Pediatric neurosurgery. 2007;43(3):236-48.

[15] Au KS, Ashley-Koch A, Northrup H. Epidemiologic and genetic aspects of spina bifida and other neural tube defects. Developmental disabilities research reviews. 2010;16(1):6-15.

[16] Schlager TA, Dilks S, Trudell J, Whittam TS, Hendley JO. Bacteriuria in children with neurogenic bladder treated with intermittent catheterization: natural history. The Journal of pediatrics. 1995 Mar 1;126(3):490-6.

[17] Worley G, Wiener JS, George TM, Fuchs HE, Mackey JF,

Fitch RD, Oldham KT. Acute abdominal symptoms and signs in children and young adults with spina bifida: Ten years' experience. Journal of pediatric surgery. 2001 Sep 1;36(9):1381-6.

[18] Wahlquist GI, McGuire E, Greene W, Herlihy E. Intermittent catheterization and urinary tract infection. Rehabilitation Nursing Journal. 1983 Jan 1;8(1):18-9.

[19] Faleiros F, Toledo C, Gomide MF, Faleiros RG, Käppler C. Right to health care and materials required for intermittent catheterization: a comparison between Germany and Brazil. Quality in Primary Care. 2015 May 1;23(3).

[20] Li LF, Leung GK, Lui WM. Sacral nerve stimulation for neurogenic bladder. World neurosurgery. 2016 Jun 1;90:236-43.

[21] Biers SM, Venn SN, Greenwell TJ. The past, present and future of augmentation cystoplasty. BJU international. 2012 May;109(9):1280-93.

[22] Küss R, Bitker M, Camey M, Chatelain C, Lassau JP. Indications and early and late results of intestino-cystoplasty: a review of 185 cases. The Journal of urology. 1970 Jan;103(1):53-63.

[23] Metcalfe PD, Casale AJ, Kaefer MA, Misseri R, Dussinger AM, Meldrum KK, Cain MP, Rink RC. Spontaneous bladder perforations: a report of 500 augmentations in children and analysis of risk. The Journal of urology. 2006 Apr;175(4):1466-71

[24] NURSE DE, Mundy AR. Assessment of the malignant potential of cystoplasty. British journal of urology. 1989 Nov;64(5):489-92.

[25] Stöhrer M, Castro-Díaz D, Chartier-Kastler E, Del Popolo G, Kramer G, Pannek J, Radziszewski P, Wyndaele JJ. Guía clínica sobre la disfunción neurógena de las vías urinarias inferiores. European Association of Urology. 2010;1:616-72.

[26] Kinnear N, Barnett D, O'Callaghan M, Horsell K, Gani J, Hennessey D. The impact of catheter-based bladder drainage method on urinary tract infection risk in spinal cord injury and neurogenic bladder: A systematic review. Neurourology and Urodynamics. 2020 Feb;39(2):854-62.

Chapter 5

Orthopedic Approach to Spina Bifida

Roselle C. Okubo, Claudio Silveri and Ana C. Belzarena

Abstract

Spina bifida is a common nervous system malformation and it encompasses a wide array of presentations with diverse orthopedic challenges. Manifestations of this disease can include dislocates hips, joint contractures, spine deformity such as scoliosis or kyphosis, clubfeet and limb rotational deformities. Additionally, many of these patients are non-ambulatory and prone to osteoporosis induced pathological fractures. The care of spina bifida patients is a challenging one, requiring many health care professionals from different areas to be working in conjunction. Nowadays, spina bifida patients live longer due to advances in health care and improving the quality of life of these patients is paramount.

Keywords: spina bifida, myelomeningocele, orthopedic surgery

1. Introduction

Spina bifida is the most common nervous system malformation. This complex disease can be considered as a group of congenital defects caused by a failure in the closure of the neural tube at the fourth week of the embryonic phase [1]. The true incidence may vary from country to country but overall is at 0.5 per 1000 births [2]. Additionally, gender prevalence is more in girls than in boys, but again it varies geographically [3]. There are mainly two categories of spina bifida, open and closed ones. The open types which include meningocele and meningomyelocele have neural tissue exposed and are more severe in terms of symptoms and prognosis [4]. Closed spina bifida or occulta, has no neural tissue exposed and includes from lipomeningocele to just a sinus tract [5]. Majority of these neural tube defects are located at lower levels of the spine, mostly in the lumbar and sacral levels [6]. These defects can be diagnosed prenatally with ultrasound imaging or maternal alpha-feto-protein levels measured on the mother's serum. Patients with spina bifida can often present with neurological deficits, motor or sensory and orthopedic conditions such as joint contractures, spine deformity, clubfeet and hip dislocations among others. The degree of the deficit and the orthopedic presentation are related to the spine level where the defect is present [4].

2. Non-orthopedic health conditions

Besides the orthopedic associated conditions, these patients can present with several other health problems. The mortality of these patients has decreased throughout the years with enhanced medical care, thus now more attention is driven at improving these patients' quality of life [7]. Intellectual disability is present only in approximately 20% of the patients and is usually the consequence of hydrocephalus [8]. Patients usually present with bladder and/or bowel incontinence, renal failure, propensity to infections and skin ulcers due to skin insensitivity, hydrocephalus, tethered cord and Arnold Chiari II type of malformation [9]. One in three of these patients will be allergic to latex, some having anaphylactic reactions. This is thought to be the consequence of repeated surgical and medical procedures, thus the importance of avoiding latex material since the beginning of care [9].

3. Pathologic fractures

Due to the lack of ambulation, physical exercise and axial bone load spina bifida patients can present with osteoporosis and osteoporosis induced fractures [10]. The

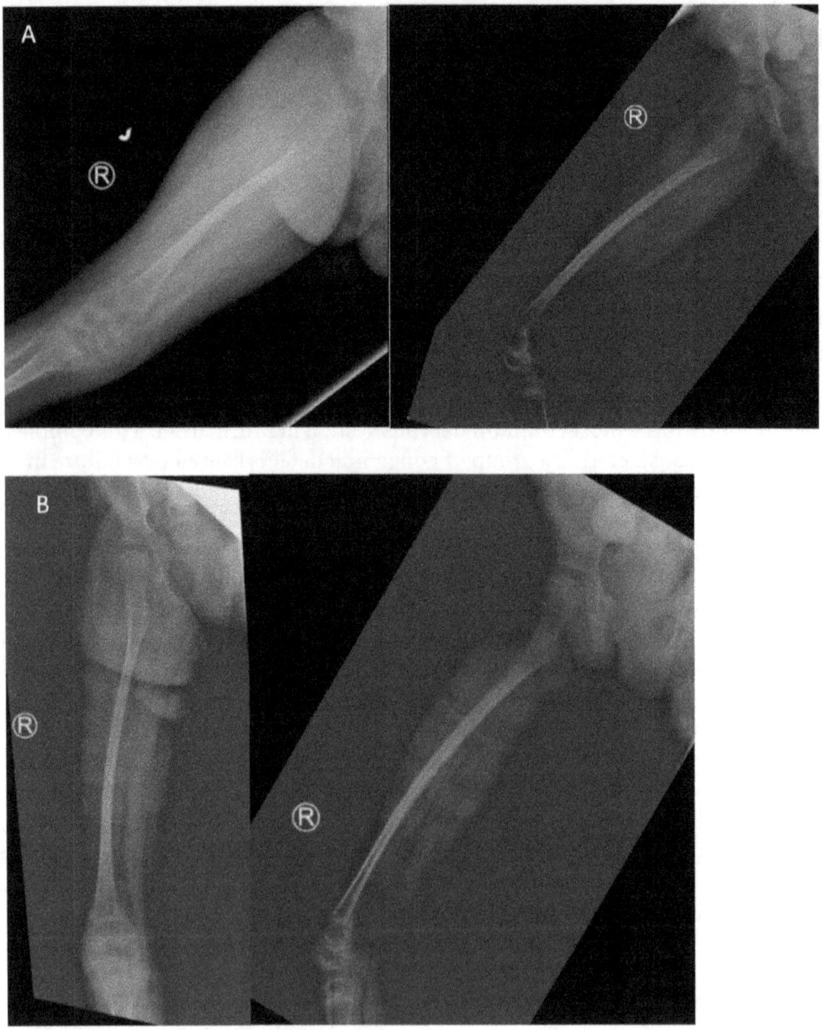

Figure 1.
Right distal femur fracture in a myelomeningocele patient without an obvious traumatic mechanism (A) and radiographic images of post-reduction and casting (B).

fractures usually occur below the neurological level of the defect and the incidence ranges from 11 to 30% [11]. The fracture mechanism is usually pathologic, these fractures usually being caused by minor trauma or even spontaneously [12]. Since many of these patients may have a fractured bone without an obvious trauma mechanism it can be difficult to diagnose these fractures. Patients usually present with a swollen, warm extremity with associated redness, and this should prompt obtaining a radiographic imaging study [13]. The caring orthopedist should be aware not to confuse these symptoms with an infection. The fractures are common the higher the level of the neural defect, in the distal femur or around the hip in patients from 3 to 7 years old (**Figure 1**) [14]. Treatment is usually non-surgical and involves immobilization in a cast. Prolonged immobilization in the cast should be minimized since this also will make osteopenia worse [15]. Patients should be assessed for bone density with dual-energy X-ray absorptiometry (DEXA scan) exams and calcium and vitamin D levels should be assessed and replaced if necessary, by the pediatrician. Weight bearing and physical exercise should be encouraged as appropriate [16].

4. Spine care

Besides the posterior element defect in the spine, spina bifida patients also present with severe congenital deformity and contractures of the spine. These deformities can pose a restriction to everyday activities as well as pulmonary function [17]. A third of the patients will have scoliosis, which is usually of an early onset and has a tendency to progress and cause pelvic obliquity [18]. Scoliosis has different causes in these patients such as muscle imbalance or primary malformations like hemivertebra and vertebral fusions. Kyphosis may also be present in approximately 15% of the patients (**Figure 2**). Is usually progressive and mostly located in the lumbar region [19]. The deformity can be so severe to cause skin breakdown at the level of the deformity (**Figure 3**). Surgery is necessary to correct the deformity and is not free of complications in these patients. Usually there is no role for bracing spine deformity in these patients and the skin insensitivity can predispose to skin ulcers and infection. Surgical correction is indicated in patients with progressing curves who are good candidates for surgery. Posterior fixation is the most common procedure performed but other options such as an anterior fusion or combined ones are used as well when appropriate. In patients with pelvic obliquity the fixation should be extended until the pelvis level, this is particularly important in non-ambulatory patients (**Figure 4**) [20]. Surgery can be associated with higher risks of infection, anesthesia complications, bleeding, non-union, hardware failure, loss

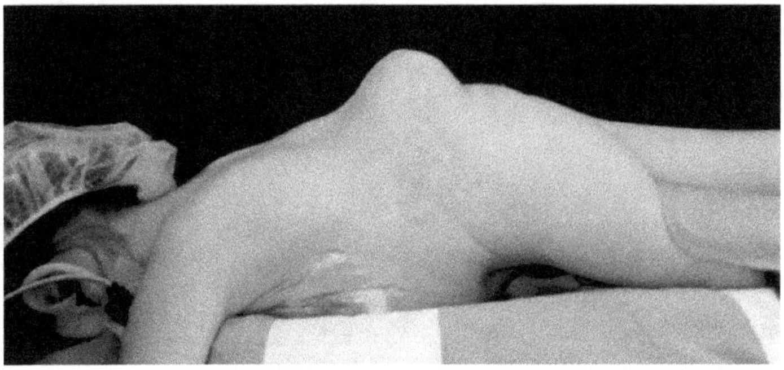

Figure 2.
Myelomeningocele patient with marked lumbar kyphosis.

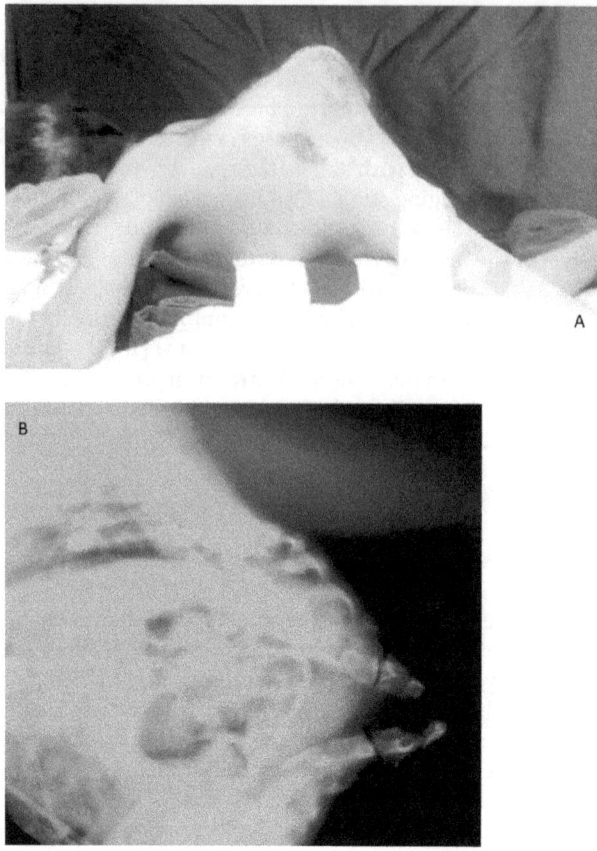

Figure 3.
Myelomeningocele patient with marked kyphosis with skin breakdown at the level of the deformity (A) and accompanying radiographic images of the deformity (B).

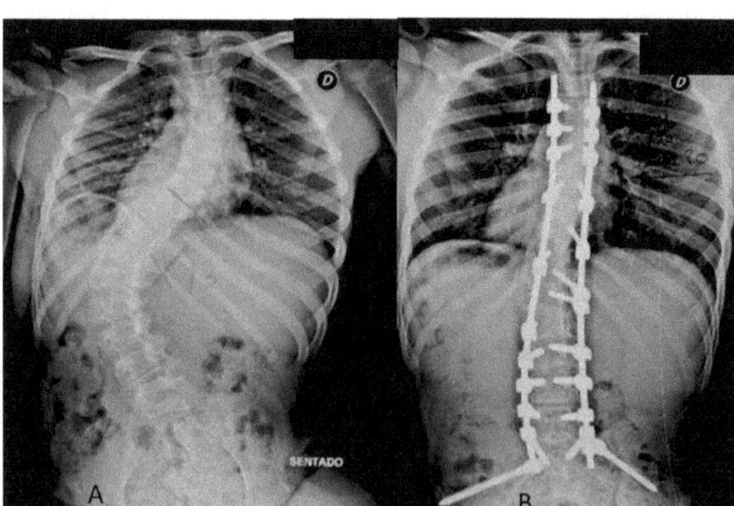

Figure 4.
Myelomeningocele patient radiographic image depicting scoliotic curve (A) and postoperative radiographic study depicting spinopelvic fusion (B).

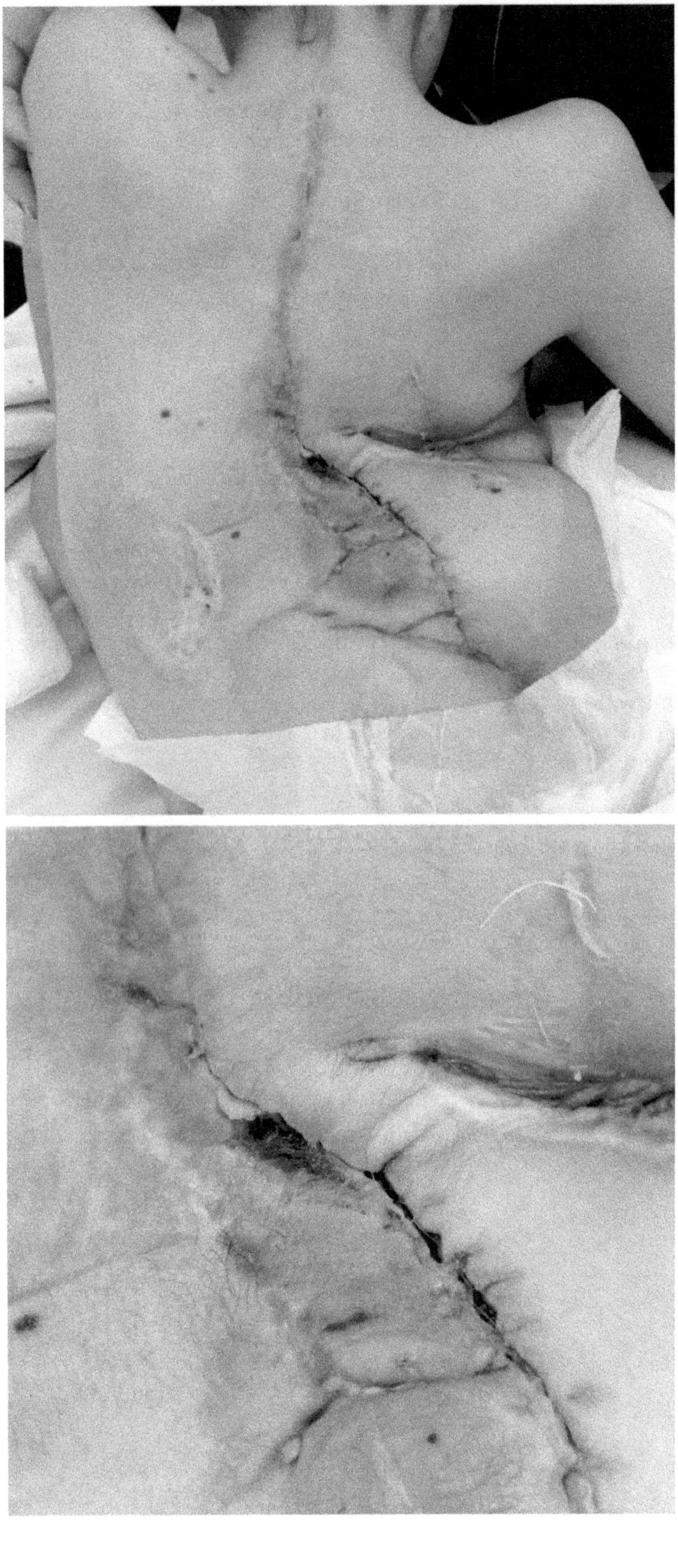

Figure 5.
Postoperative skin breakdown and infection in a myelomeningocele patient.

of correction, pressure sores, subsequent operations and even death (**Figure 5**) [21]. Some studies have suggested a higher rate of union when using a combined anterior and posterior approach [22].

Another spine problem spina bifida patients may present with is tethered cord syndrome. This occurs when the spinal cord is stretched because it remains attached distally, usually to scar tissue from prior surgical procedures. Most patients have some degree of cord tethering but only 30% manifest clinically. Patients who have symptoms present with progressive scoliosis, new gait abnormalities or changes, weakness, spasticity or back pain [23]. Neurosurgeons are the specialists who treat this problem surgically by untethering the cord.

5. Hip

Thirty percent of the spina bifida patients present with hip dislocations either at birth or during their childhood (**Figure 6**) [24]. The number can go up to 50% if we include hip subluxations. Dislocation occurs more commonly when the spinal cord defect is at the L3 level and the patient has a muscle imbalance with unopposed hip flexion and adduction. The ability of a patient to walk does not seem to be affected by dislocation of the hips and surgical relocation does not necessarily translate in a functional improvement [25]. Additionally, this problem does not seem to cause pain to the patients. For all these reasons many orthopedic surgeons advocate against putting the patients through complex osseous and soft tissue procedures and surgical intervention can even be considered controversial in such scenario where a benefit will not necessarily be obtained and such interventions are not exempt from surgical complications [26, 27].

6. Knee deformities

The most common knee problems spina bifida patients present with are knee flexion contracture and knee extension contracture [13]. Less commonly valgus deformity and instability [27]. There are many causes for those deformities such as muscle imbalance, fibrosis of the surrounding tissues and eventually a fracture malunion. A flexion contracture can usually be present at birth, different form

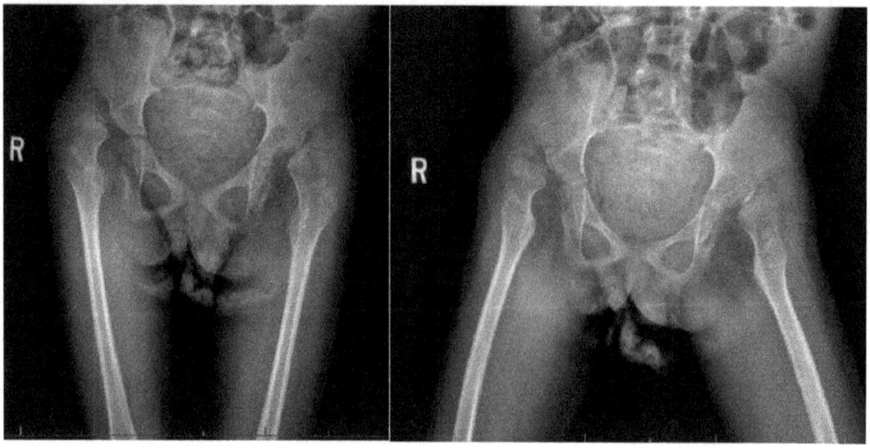

Figure 6.
Bilateral hip dislocation and osteopenia in a 14-years-old patient with spina bifida.

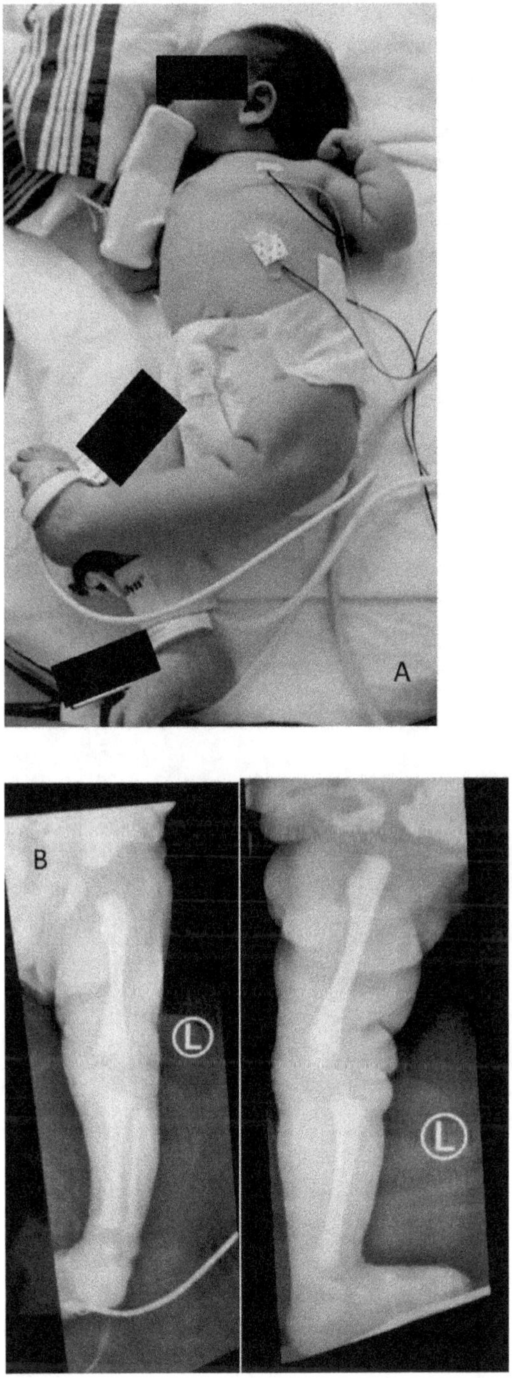

Figure 7.
Newborn with congenital knee dislocation in extension (A) and front and lateral radiographic image depicting the knee extension deformity (B).

the flexed knee found in healthy newborns, in myelomeningocele patients this deformity is fixed and more difficult to treat. The higher the level of the spinal cord defect the more severe is the knee contracture [28]. Patient positioning and muscle imbalance are thought to be involved in the genesis of this deformity. If the patient is non-ambulatory the fixed knee flexion contracture does not cause any functional impairment, but in ambulatory patients it should be addressed. Surgical treatment is indicated when the flexion contracture is >20 degrees [29]. Treatment usually involves the releasing of the surrounding soft tissues such as hamstrings, gastrocnemius and posterior capsule. In more severe cases and usually in older patients an extension osteotomy may be indicated as well [30].

Knee extension is also usually present at birth, usually bilateral and much less common than the flexion contracture (**Figure** 7). The treating orthopedic surgeon should be aware of other associated deformities such as ipsilateral hip dislocation, external hip contracture and equinovarus foot [31]. If the patient presents with

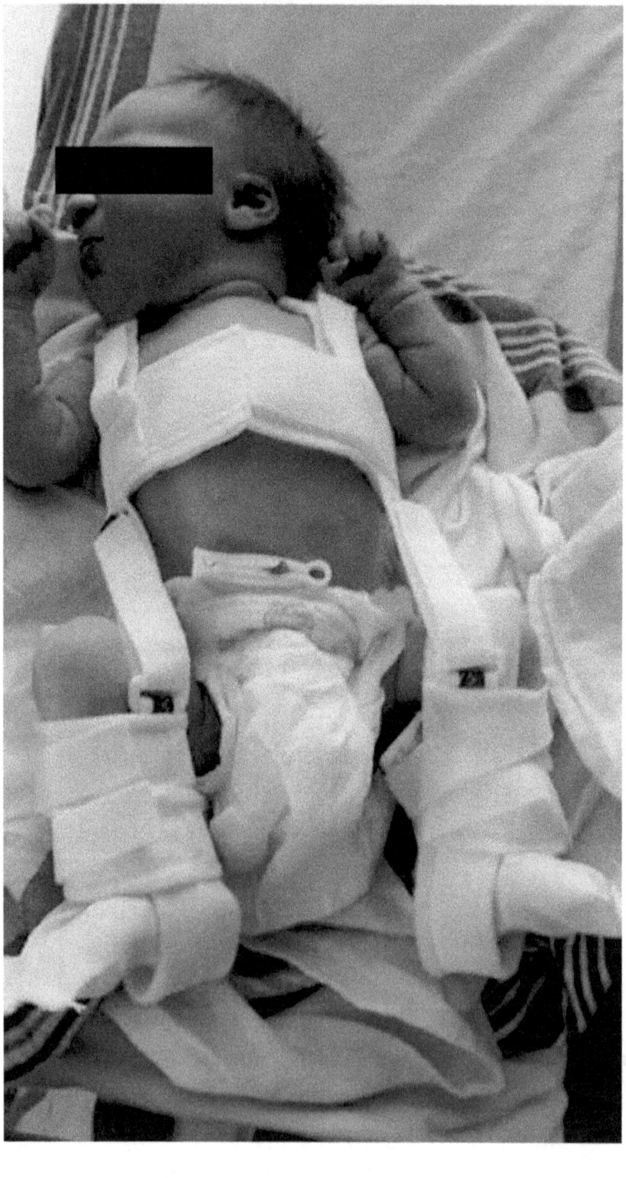

Figure 8.
Newborn wearing a Pavlik harness, the harness requires the knee to be bendable in order to fit appropriately.

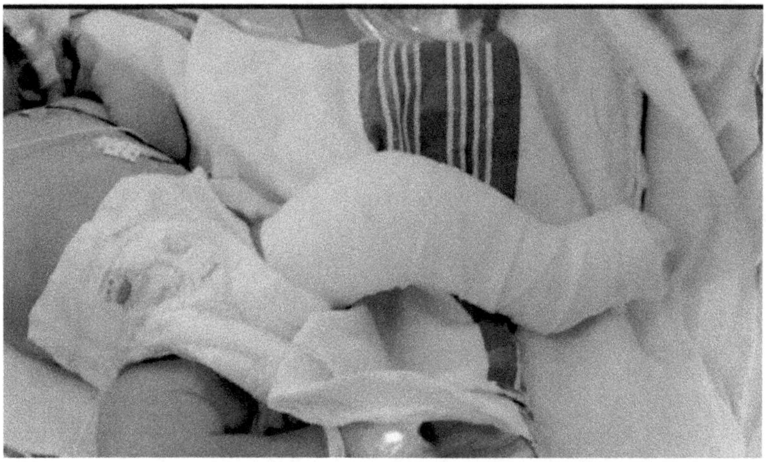

Figure 9.
Extension deformity being treated by serial casting aiming a achieving a 90 degrees knee flexion.

hip dislocation and knee extension deformity simultaneously at birth, the knee deformity should be addressed first, so that the newborn can afterwards, once the knee deformity has been corrected, wear a Pavlik harness to treat the hip dislocation (**Figure 8**) [32]. The treatment for the knee extension deformity consists in serial casting until a 90 degree flexion is achieved (**Figure 9**). The treating orthopedic surgeon should be aware of not utilizing much force to flex the knee since the distal femur can be bent and even fractured in extreme cases. Casting should be followed by physical therapy. In resistant cases where casting is not successful surgical intervention is indicated. The surgical procedure usually consists of V-Y quadriceps lengthening and anterior capsulotomy [33].

7. Foot deformities

Foot and ankle deformity are very prevalent in spina bifida patients, with an incidence ranging from 60 to 90%. They can be present at birth or developed later on in life in close relationship with the spinal defect level [34]. In addition to the muscle imbalance and deformity the patients present with insensate feet which places a risk for skin breakdown and infections. The most common foot deformities are calcaneus, equinus, Varus, valgus, clubfeet and vertical talus and they can present as a single deformity or in combination [35]. Treatment of foot and ankle deformities is aimed at achieving a braceable plantigrade foot. In general treatment may start with casting or bracing and potentially a soft tissue surgical intervention to avoid fixed bone deformities. Once those are present osteotomies are needed to correct the foot. The patient needs to be examined regularly by a specialized pediatric orthopedist to detect tightness and incipient deformities can be early addressed (**Figure 10**).

7.1 Clubfoot

Spina bifida patients present with a rigid clubfoot deformity that is in general resistant to casting. This type of deformity can occur in up to 30–50% of the patients and the frequency increases with higher levels of the spine defect [36]. Casting with the Ponseti technique should be attempted and even though most of the patients achieve correction by this method almost 70% will relapse [37].

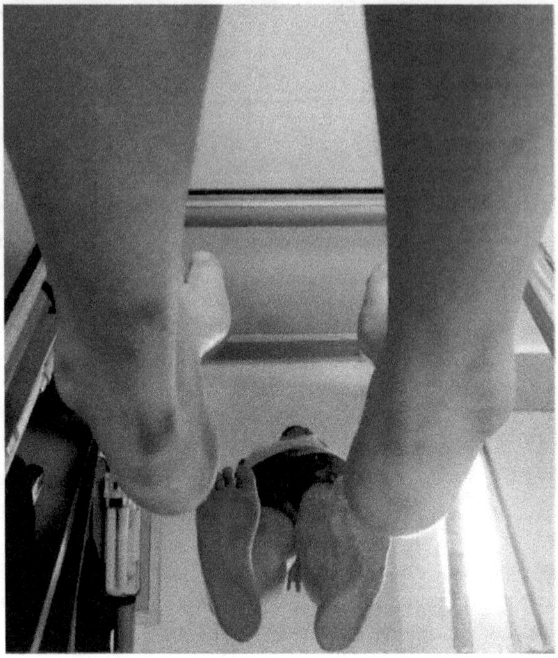

Figure 10.
Patient with a bilateral cavovarus deformity being examined in clinic with the help of a podoscope.

Additionally, if serial casting is being implement is paramount to assess skin integrity at every cast change in these patients due to their insensate feet. After correction is achieved by casting the treatment is followed by an Achilles tendon tenotomy, usually open in these patients [38]. If a wider soft tissue release is needed later on due to a recurrence a radical posteromedial release is recommended. In this procedure the subtalar, talonavicular and calcaneocuboid joints are completely released. After surgery casting followed by ankle foot orthosis (AFO) is required to maintain the correction. If a recurrence is then again noted, which may occur in 20–50% of the patients, a talectomy is indicated to achieve a plantigrade braceable foot [39].

7.2 Equinus

This deformity is also associated with higher levels of spina bifida. If the deformity is flexible an AFO may be attempted to prevent further progressing to a rigid equinus (**Figure 11**). With increasing severity of the deformity an Achilles tendon excision is recommended and even a radical posterior release if a plantigrade foot is not achieved after the Achilles resection [40]. Once the foot is an acceptable position a K wire is used in the talocalcaneal joint to maintain the alignment while to foot remains in a cast for at least 6 weeks (**Figure 12**).

7.3 Cavovarus

Cavovarus foot deformity is more prevalent in patients with a sacral level spina bifida and it is present in up to 17% of the patients [41]. The deformity is the cause of foot muscle imbalance (**Figure 13**). The treatment is dependent on how flexible the hindfoot is. This must be assessed by the orthopedic surgeon with the Coleman

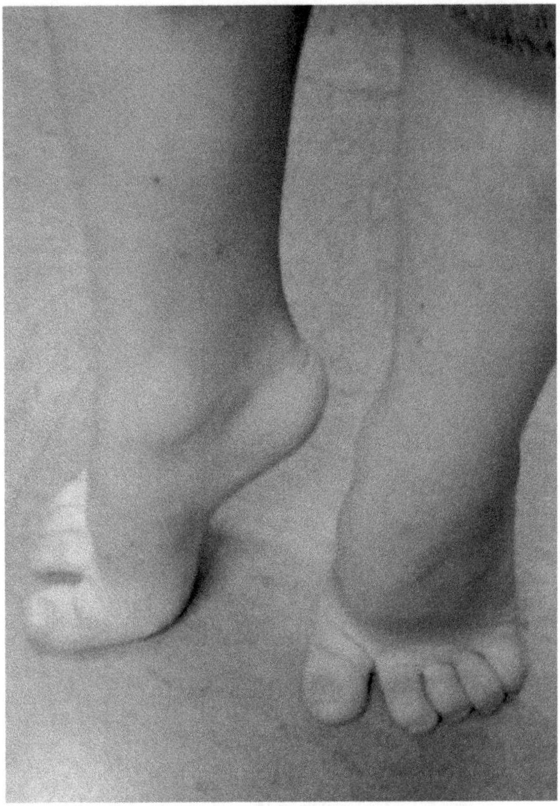

Figure 11.
Four-year-old patient with bilateral equinus.

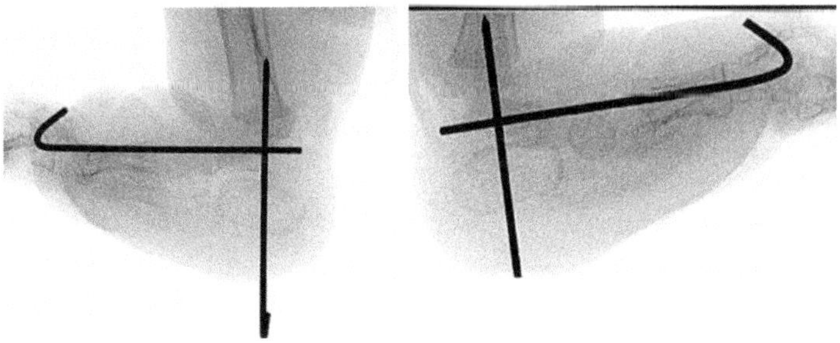

Figure 12.
K wires used after posterior release in a 12 months old patient with rigid bilateral clubfeet.

block test. If the hindfoot is flexible, only the forefoot will need to be addressed surgically. Meanwhile on the case of a rigid hindfoot several osteotomies may be needed to achieve correction. The current recommendations with high percent of success are for a first metatarsal closing wedge, an opening plantar wedge osteotomy of the medial cuneiform, a closing wedge cuboid osteotomy and sliding calcaneus osteotomy [42, 43].

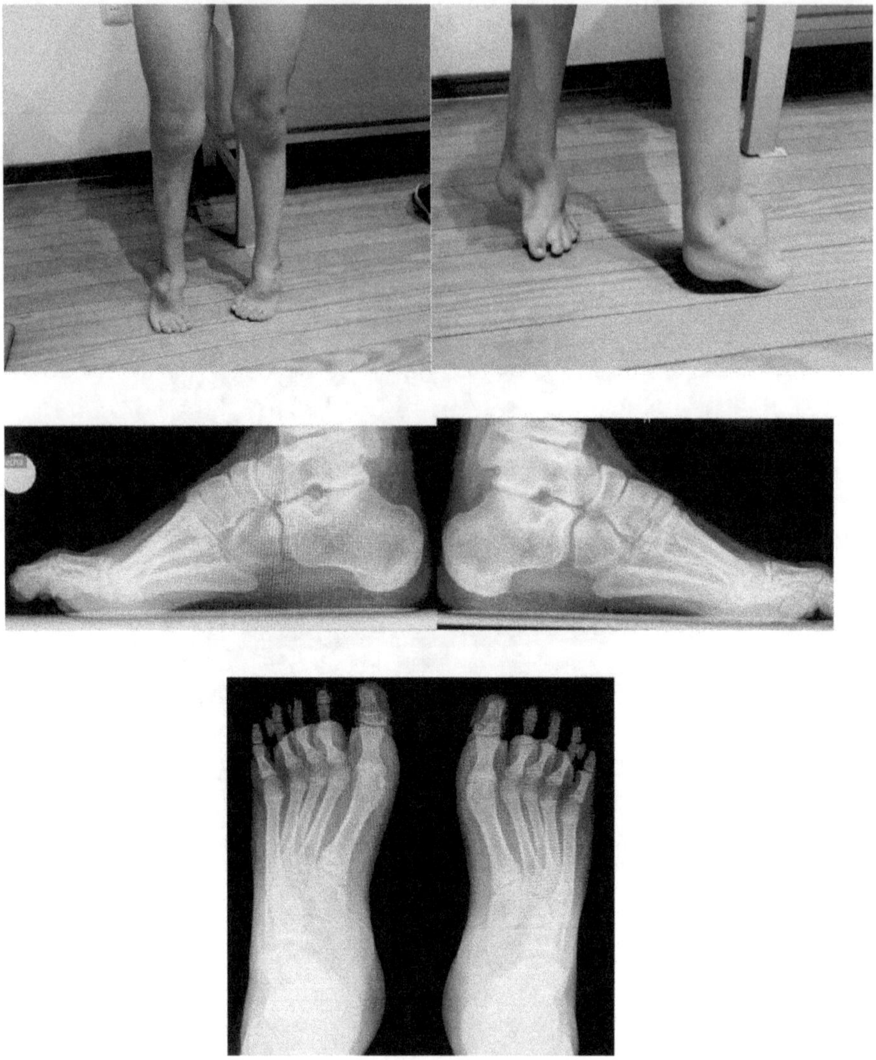

Figure 13.
Myelomeningocele patient with bilateral cavovarus feet and accompanying radiographic images depicting the high medial arch and the varus deformity.

8. Conclusions

Spina Bifida comprehends a complex subset of congenital malformation with a wide array of clinical presentation and truly diverse challenges to the patients affected by it. It is paramount that a team of multiple health care professionals from several areas of specialty work together to help improve the outcomes and life quality of these patients. The orthopedic surgeon is usually involved shortly after birth and continues to follow spina bifida patients for long terms into adulthood.

Conflict of interest

The authors state no conflict of interest related to the writing of this chapter.

Author details

Roselle C. Okubo[1], Claudio Silveri[2] and Ana C. Belzarena[1]*

1 Pediatric Orthopedic Service, Baptist Health South Florida, Miami, Florida, United States

2 Pediatric Orthopedics Service, University of the Republic, Montevideo, Uruguay

*Address all correspondence to: ceciliabel@baptisthealth.net

References

[1] Feeley BT, Ip TC, Otsuka NY. Skeletal maturity in myelomeningocele. Journal of Pediatric Orthopedics. 2003;**23**(6):718-721

[2] Parker SE, Mai CT, Canfield MA, et al. Updated national birth prevalence estimates for selected birth defects in the United States, 2004-2006. Birth Defects Research Part A: Clinical and Molecular Teratology. 2010;**88**(12):1008-1016

[3] Mitchell LE, Adzick NS, Melchionne J, Pasquariello PS, Sutton LN, Whitehead AS. Spina bifida. Lancet. 2004;**364**(9448):1885-1895

[4] Jobe AH. Fetal surgery for myelomeningocele. The New England Journal of Medicine. 2002;**347**(4):230-231

[5] Iskandar BJ, Fulmer BB, Hadley MN, Oakes WJ. Congenital tethered spinal cord syndrome in adults. Journal of Neurosurgery. 1998;**88**(6):958-961

[6] Sutton LN. Fetal surgery for neural tube defects. Best Practice and Research Clinical Obstetrics and Gynaecology. 2008;**22**(1):175-188

[7] Bowman RM, McLone DG, Grant JA, Tomita T, Ito JA. Spina bifida outcome: A 25-year prospective. Pediatric Neurosurgery. 2001;**34**(3):114-120

[8] Fletcher JM et al. Spinal lesion level in spina bifida: A source of neural and cognitive heterogeneity. Journal of Neurosurgery. 2005;**268-279**(PubMed: 15881750):102

[9] Verhoef M, Barf HA, Post MWM, van Asbeck FWA, Gooskens RHJM, Prevo AJH. Functional independence among young adults with spina bifida, in relation to hydrocephalus and level of lesion. Developmental Medicine and Child Neurology. 2006;**48**(2):114-119

[10] Anschuetz RH, Freehafer AA, Shaffer JW, Dixon Jr. MS. Severe fracture complications in myelodysplasia. Journal of Pediatric Orthopedics 1984; 4(1):22-24.

[11] Marreiros H, Monteiro L, Loff C, Calado E. Fractures in children and adolescents with spina bifida – Experience of a portuguese tertiary care hospital. Developmental Medicine and Child Neurology. 2010;**52**(8):754-759

[12] Okurowska-Zawada B, Konstantynowicz J, Kulak W, Kaczmarski M, Piotrowska-Jastrzebska J, Sienkiewicz D, et al. Assessment of risks factors for osteoporosis and fractures in children with meningomyelocele. Advances in Medical Sciences. 2009;**54**(2):247-252

[13] Westcott, M. A., Dynes, M. C., Remer, E. M., Donaldson, J. S., & Dias, L. S. (1992). Congenital and acquired orthopedic abnormalities in patients with myelomeningocele. Radiographics, 12(6), 1155-1173. doi:10.1148/radiographics.12.6.1439018.

[14] Kumar, S. J., Cowell, H. R., & Townsend, P. (1984). Physeal, metaphyseal, and Diaphyseal injuries of the lower extremities in children with myelomeningocele. Journal of Pediatric Orthopaedics, 4(1), 25-27. doi:10.1097/01241398-198401000-00006

[15] Korhonen BJ. Fractures in myelodysplasia. Clinical Orthopaedics and Related Research. 1971;**79**:145-155

[16] Shaw NJ. Management of osteoporosis in children. European Journal of Endocrinology. 2008;**159**:S33-S39

[17] Banta JV, Park SM. Improvement in pulmonary function in patients having combined anterior and posterior spine

fusion for myelomeningocele scoliosis. Spine (Phila Pa 1976). 1983;**8**:765-770

[18] Drennan JC. The role of muscles in the development of human lumbar kyphosis. Developmental Medicine & Child Neurology. 2008;*12*:33-38. DOI: 10.1111/j.1469-8749.1970.tb03000.x

[19] Asher M, Olson J. Factors affecting the ambulatory status of patients with spina bifida cystica. The Journal of Bone and Joint Surgery. American Volume. 1983;**65**:350-356

[20] Bulman, W. A., Dormans, J. P., Ecker, M. L., & Drummond, D. S. (1996). Posterior spinal fusion for scoliosis in patients with cerebral palsy: A comparison of Luque rod and unit rod instrumentation. Journal of Pediatric Orthopaedics, 314-323. doi:10.1097/00004694-199605000-00005.

[21] Banit DM, Iwinski HJ Jr, Talwalkar V, Johnson M. Posterior spinal fusion in paralytic scoliosis and myelomeningocele. Journal of Pediatric Orthopedics. 2001;**21**:117-125

[22] Osebold WR, Mayfield JK, Winter RB, Moe JH. Surgical treatment of paralytic scoliosis associated with myelomeningocele. The Journal of Bone and Joint Surgery. American Volume. 1982;**64**:841-856

[23] Sarwark JF, Weber DT, Gabrieli AP, Mclone DG, Dias L. Tethered cord syndrome in low motor level children with myelomeningocele. In: *Spina Bifida*. 1999. pp. 128-130. DOI: 10.1007/978-4-431-68373-5_27

[24] Broughton NS, Menelaus MB, Cole WG, Shurtleff DB. The natural history of hip deformity in myelomeningocele. Journal of Bone and Joint Surgery. British Volume (London). 1993;**75**:760-763

[25] Canale G, Scarsi M, Mastragostino S. Hip deformity and dislocation in spina bifida. Italian Journal of Orthopaedics and Traumatology. 1992;**18**(2):155-165

[26] Sherk HH, Uppal GS, Lane G, Melchionni J. Treatment versus non-treatment of hip dislocations in ambulatory patients with myelomeningocele. Developmental Medicine and Child Neurology. 1991;**33**(6):491-494

[27] Swaroop VT, Dias LS. Strategies of hip management in myelomeningocele: To do or not to do. Hip International. 2009;**19**(Suppl 6):S53-S55

[28] Dias LS. Myelomeningocele and intraspinal lipoma. In: Sponseller PD, editor. Orthopaedic Knowledge Update: Pediatrics 2nd Edn. American Academy of Orthopaedic Surgeons. 2002. pp. 249-259

[29] Dias LS. Surgical management of knee contractures in myelomeningocele. Journal of Pediatric Orthopedics. 1982 Jun;**2**(2):127-131

[30] Moen T, Gryfakis N, Dias L, Lemke L. Crouched gait in myelomeningocele: A comparison between the degree of knee flexion contracture in the clinical examination and during gait. Journal of Pediatric Orthopedics. 2005;**25**(5):657-660. DOI: 10.1097/01.mph.0000165136.76238.23

[31] Herring J. Neuromuscular disorders. In: Tachdjian's pediatric orthopaedics. Saunders Elsevier (2008), Philadelphia, pp 1405-1453.

[32] Tosi LL, Buck BD, Nason SS, McKay DW. Dislocation of hip in myelomeningocele. The McKay hip stabilization. The Journal of Bone and Joint Surgery. American Volume. 1996;**78**(5):664-673. DOI: 10.2106/00004623-199605000-00005

[33] Curtis BH, Fisher RL. Congenital hyperextension with anterior

subluxation of the knee. Surgical treatment and long-term observations. The Journal of Bone and Joint Surgery. American Volume. 1969;**51**(2):255-269

[34] Noonan KJ, Didelot WP, Lindseth RE. Care of the pediatric foot in myelodysplasia. Foot and Ankle Clinics. 2000;**5**(2):281-304

[35] Maynard MJ, Weiner LS, Burke SW. Neuropathic foot ulceration in patients with myelodysplasia. Journal of Pediatric Orthopedics. 1992;**12**:786-788

[36] Flynn JM, Herrera-Soto JA, Ramirez NF, Fernandez-Feliberti R, Vilella F, Guzman J. Clubfoot release in myelodysplasia. Journal of Pediatric Orthopaedics. Part B. 2004;**13**:259-262

[37] Gerlach DJ, Gurnett CA, Limpaphayom N, Alaee F, Zhang Z, Porter K, et al. Early results of the Ponseti method for the treatment of clubfoot associated with myelomeningocele. The Journal of Bone and Joint Surgery. American Volume. 2009;**91**(6):1350-1359

[38] Swaroop VT, Dias L. Orthopaedic management of spina bifida—Part II: Foot and ankle deformities. Journal of Children's Orthopaedics. 2011;5(6):403-414. DOI: 10.1007/s11832-011-0368-9

[39] Dias LS, Stern LS. Talectomy in the treatment of resistant talipes equinovarus deformity in myelomeningocele and arthrogryposis. Journal of Pediatric Orthopedics. 1987;7:39-41

[40] Sharrard WJ, Grosfield I. The management of deformity and paralysis of the foot in myelomeningocele. Journal of Bone and Joint Surgery. British Volume (London). 1968;**50**:456-465

[41] Frawley PA, Broughton NS, Menelaus MB. Incidence and type of hindfoot deformities in patients with low-level spina bifida. Journal of Pediatric Orthopedics. 1998;**18**:312-313

[42] Mubarak SJ, Van Valin SE. Osteotomies of the foot for cavus deformities in children. Journal of Pediatric Orthopedics. 2009;**29**(3):294-299

[43] Schwend RM, Drennan JC. Cavus foot deformity in children. The Journal of the American Academy of Orthopaedic Surgeons. 2003;**11**:201-211

Section 2

Craniosynostosis

Chapter 6

New Technologies to Improve Surgical Outcome during Open-Cranial Vault Remodeling

David García-Mato, Javier Pascau and Santiago Ochandiano

Abstract

Current approaches for the surgical correction of craniosynostosis are highly dependent on surgeon experience. Therefore, outcomes are often inadequate, causing suboptimal esthetic results. Novel methods for cranial shape analysis based on statistical shape models enable accurate and objective diagnosis from preoperative 3D photographs or computed tomography scans. Moreover, advanced algorithms are now available to calculate a reference cranial shape for each patient from a multi-atlas of healthy cases, and to determine the most optimal approach to restore normal calvarial shape. During surgery, multiple technologies are available to ensure accurate translation of the preoperative virtual plan into the operating room. Patient-specific cutting guides and templates can be designed and manufactured to assist during osteotomy and remodeling. Then, intraoperative navigation and augmented reality visualization can provide real-time guidance during the placement and fixation of the remodeled bone. Finally, 3D photography enables intraoperative surgical outcome evaluation and postoperative patient follow-up. This chapter summarizes recent literature on all these technologies, showing how their integration into the surgical workflow could increase reproducibility and reduce inter-surgeon variability in open cranial vault remodeling procedures.

Keywords: craniosynostosis, surgery, shape analysis, computer-assisted planning, outcome evaluation

1. Introduction

Craniosynostosis is a birth defect defined as the premature closure of one or more cranial sutures [1]. Compensatory growth of the brain along the non-fused sutures produces morphological abnormalities, including dysmorphic cranial vault and facial asymmetry, which can lead to severe conditions such as increased intracranial pressure and impaired brain growth [2]. Prevalence studies indicate that craniosynostosis affects 1 of every 2000–2500 live births worldwide [3, 4].

Although the management of craniosynostosis has significantly improved, surgical correction is the preferred approach for treatment in most cases. The objective of surgical correction is to release the fused suture and to normalize calvarial shape. Minimally invasive techniques (endoscopic, linear craniectomy) have been proposed as an alternative to open surgery [5]. These procedures are usually followed by postoperative helmet-molding therapy to facilitate appropriate changes in the cranial morphology [6]. However, these limited approaches are typically reserved for the treatment of mild-to-moderate deformities affecting young patients (less than 6 months old) [2].

The rest of the cases are commonly treated through open cranial vault remodeling, which aims to normalize the calvarial shape to increase intracranial volume and reduce the risk of elevated intracranial pressure. Typical cranial vault remodeling begins with a coronal incision to allow exposure of the calvarial surface. Then, osteotomy of multiple segments in the affected bone region is performed and the different fragments are reconfigured to achieve a normal cranial morphology. Finally, the remodeled bone fragments are transferred to the patient and rigidly fixed and secured using resorbable plates [7, 8]. This operation is typically performed before the first year of life to maximize reossification and to benefit from the malleability of the bone tissue [9].

Distraction osteogenesis is an alternative surgical approach for the treatment of craniosynostosis, which has been accepted by many surgeons [10]. This technique involves the application of graduated tension to the bone tissue using external fixation devices. The main advantage of this procedure is the reduced invasiveness in comparison with open cranial vault remodeling, since the dissection of the dura is limited [11]. However, it shows limitations such as long treatment duration and, in some cases, secondary surgical interventions.

Nowadays, diagnosis and surgical correction of craniosynostosis are still highly dependent on the subjective assessment and artistic judgment of surgeons [12]. They must determine the degree of the deformity and the best approach for remodeling of the cranial vault to restore normal calvarial shape. As a result, there exists a high variability in the performance of surgeons and, thus, in the surgical outcomes. Although optimal surgical results may be achieved by the more experienced craniofacial surgeons, more complications may arise among the less experienced. Several studies, evaluating the long-term postoperative results after surgical correction between 1987 and 2013, have reported complication rates varying between 2% and 23.3%, and reoperation rates as high as 10–36% [13–19]. In addition, these studies reported that between 9.9% and 36% of the patients presented moderate-to-severe malformations after surgical treatment, causing suboptimal esthetic outcomes (Whitaker class III/IV).

Therefore, there is a clinical need to improve the reproducibility of surgical outcomes and to reduce intersurgeon variability in craniosynostosis surgery. Multiple technological advancements are now available to improve diagnosis, preoperative planning, surgical performance, and postoperative evaluation of craniosynostosis patients. However, recent literature presenting and comparing alternative technologies to assist during craniosynostosis surgery is not available and, as a result, craniofacial surgeons may not be aware of these advances. This chapter aims to provide an overview of the different developments in the field of craniosynostosis through a detailed review and analysis of the literature.

2. Cranial shape analysis and diagnosis

Although the fusion of sutures is a clear indication of craniosynostosis in most cases, an evaluation of the cranial shape abnormality is crucial to determine the need for surgical correction. However, there are no objective methods available in the clinical practice to quantify cranial malformations, making the diagnosis and the virtual surgical planning highly dependent on the surgeon's expertise [20].

The analysis of the preoperative morphology is the most critical step when planning surgery [21]. A 3D volumetric evaluation of the patient's anatomy in comparison with normal morphology is essential to comprehend the basis of the cranial malformations and to determine the best approach for surgical correction. In this context, several methods based on statistical shape models have been proposed to objectify diagnosis and planning in craniosynostosis. The idea of these approaches is to define the normal cranial shape from a dataset of healthy subjects and to compare it with the pathological shape of the subject under evaluation to provide a patient-specific diagnosis and reference for planning.

Saber et al. [22] generated a library of normative pediatric skulls from computed tomography (CT) scans of 103 healthy subjects. Each CT scan was segmented, and a set of reference points was distributed onto the outer surface of the skull. Then, all 3D models were aligned and an average composite skull, "super-skull", was created from the data of all 103 patients providing an estimation of what a normal child skull looks like. For each new subject with craniosynostosis, the composite skull model can be scaled to their age and head circumference to obtain an appropriate normative reference for that subject. This approach requires age stratification and suffers from the limitation of defining landmark correspondence.

Later, Mendoza et al. [23] presented a statistical shape model of normal anatomy constructed via principal component analysis (PCA). Each new subject under study is projected into the PCA shape space and its closest normal cranial shape is computed through similarity metrics in the PCA space. Moreover, age-invariance is achieved using a registration algorithm that aligns and scales the subject's cranial shape with the reference normal shape only considering the anatomy at the base of the skull, where pathological deformations during craniosynostosis are negligible [24]. This methodology presents an improvement in comparison with previous approaches [22, 25], which were based on population averages or age-matched templates, and accounts for normal variations in healthy anatomy (e.g. due to sex or ethnicity [26]).

Comparison of the cranial shape of a patient with its closest normal reference, computed from statistical shape models, can be used to discriminate pathological shape abnormalities from healthy phenotypes. The malformation field for each subject can be computed by measuring the Euclidean distance from each vertex of the subject's skull surface model to the closest vertex in the most similar normal model. Local malformation values in the different regions of the cranium can then be visualized using a color map (**Figure 1**).

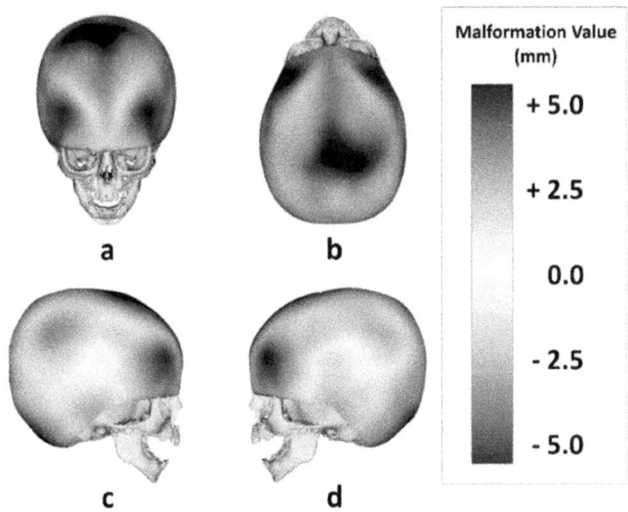

Figure 1.
Malformation field of a patient with metopic craniosynostosis computed by comparing the preoperative cranial shape with its closest normal reference: (a) anterior view, (b) superior view, (c) right view, and (d) left view.

Malformation fields provide valuable information on the degree of morphological abnormality and can be used for automatic diagnosis. Mendoza et al. [27] used a dataset of 18 patients with metopic craniosynostosis to identify three robust landmarks for diagnosis and characterization of trigonocephaly. The malformation field for each patient in the dataset was averaged across metopic craniosynostosis subjects and represented on a template of normal anatomy. Then, optimal landmarks were defined on the points of maximum average malformation on the frontal bone region. Wood et al. [28] demonstrated that the interfrontal angle value, measured using these three optimal landmarks, presented significantly different values in metopic craniosynostosis patients and healthy phenotypes. They obtained an accuracy of 98% for the diagnosis of metopic synostosis using this methodology. Similar approaches have been proposed for the quantification of other types of craniosynostosis, such as unicoronal [29] or sagittal [30].

3D reconstructions generated from CT scans are the basis of most methods for quantitative evaluation of cranial shape. This imaging technique has become the standard for the investigation of potential craniosynostosis due to its ability to display bone tissue with high spatial resolution [31]. CT imaging enables the generation of accurate 3D reconstructions of the cranium which can be used for diagnosis, shape analysis, and virtual surgical planning. However, this technique involves the exposure of the infants to ionizing radiation and frequently requires sedation or anesthesia. For these reasons, CT imaging is rarely used for postoperative evaluation of surgical outcomes and patient follow-up [32].

Due to the limitations of CT imaging, 3D photography has been introduced for the evaluation of cranial malformations. The validity and reliability of this technology to obtain craniofacial anthropometric measurements have already been demonstrated [33–35]. In particular, Porras et al. [36] showed how 3D photography discriminates between patients with and without craniosynostosis with a sensitivity

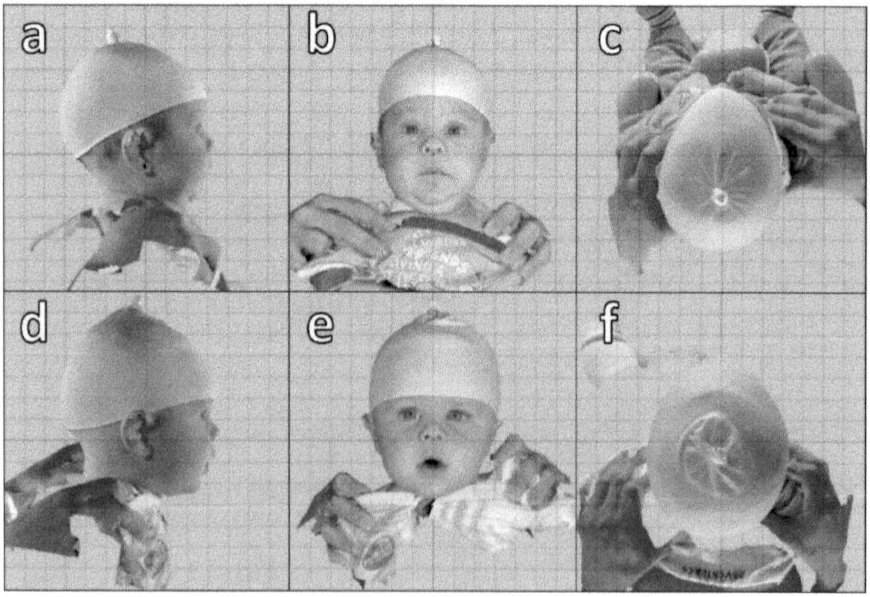

Figure 2.
Preoperative (a-c) and postoperative (d-f) 3D photographs of a metopic craniosynostosis patient. The patient's hair covered using a skull cap to avoid artifacts. Image adapted from [35].

above 94%. Other authors have shown that it is possible to calculate intracranial volume with this technique [37].

3D photography followed by statistical shape analysis provides a powerful tool for fast, non-invasive, and radiation-free quantification of cranial shape, presenting a valuable alternative to CT imaging. This technology enables the visualization and quantification of global and regional cranial malformations without exposure to ionizing radiation. Besides, the acquisition of 3D photographs is very fast, avoiding the need for sedation or anesthesia of the infant. Multiple 3D photographs can be acquired for diagnosis and postoperative evaluation of the surgical outcomes. The main limitation of 3D photography is the difficulty in capturing hair. This issue is easily solved by covering the patient's hair during the acquisition using tight nylon skull caps to avoid artifacts (**Figure 2**) [38]. A suboptimal covering of the hair may cause bumps on the surface that will affect cranial shape quantification.

Cranial shape analysis can provide an objective and accurate diagnosis of craniosynostosis. This tool can eliminate subjectivity and increase reproducibility during the diagnostic phase. The integration of these advancements in the clinical practice will contribute to the early diagnosis of craniosynostosis, which is crucial for management, prevention of complications, and consideration for prompt surgical correction [39].

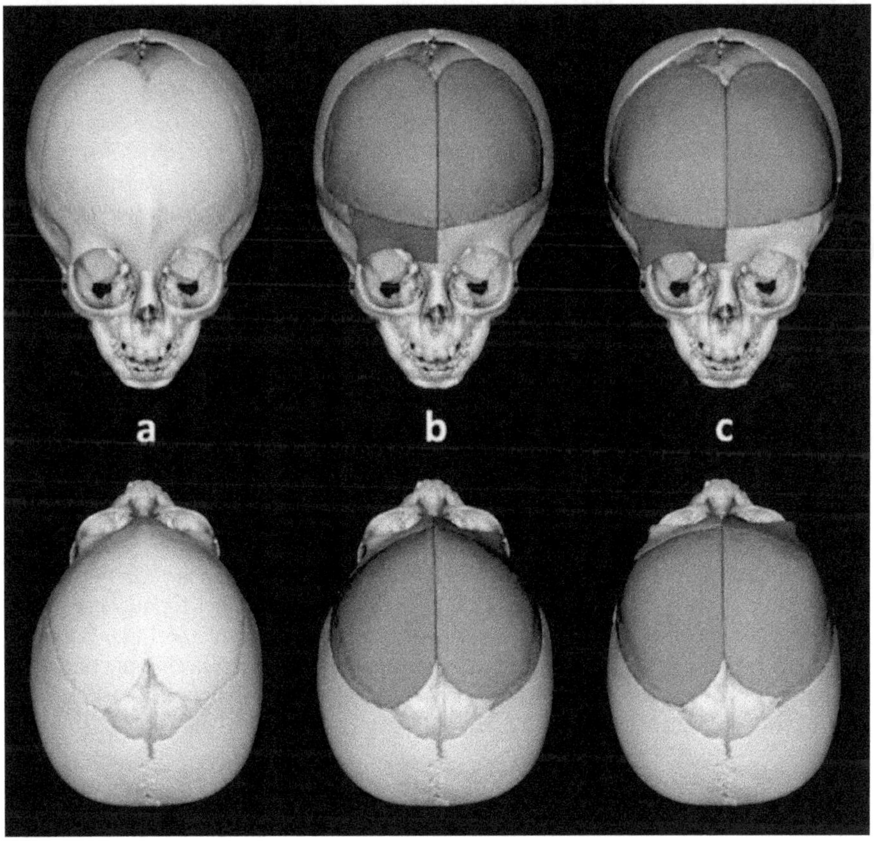

Figure 3.
Virtual surgical plan of open cranial vault remodeling for correction of metopic craniosynostosis: (a) 3D model of the cranium obtained from preoperative CT scan, (b) definition of osteotomy lines and fragments, and (c) configuration of bone fragments to achieve desired postoperative cranial shape.

3. Computer-assisted planning

Once a patient is diagnosed with craniosynostosis, surgical correction is the standard of care for most moderate to severe deformities. During the surgical procedure, surgeons perform a remodeling of the affected region to create a normal cranial shape. However, "normal" cranial shape is usually defined through mental constructions by experienced craniofacial surgeons, and is thus highly subjective. Therefore, determining the best approach to restore normal shape remains a subjective surgical art, leading to a less reliable prediction of the surgical outcome of each patient.

Computer-assisted surgical planning has been proposed to enhance the accuracy, efficiency, and reproducibility of craniosynostosis surgeries [21, 40]. Virtual surgery can be performed preoperatively on a computer workstation to reduce time-consuming intraoperative decision making. During virtual planning, osteotomies are defined and bone fragments are configured to achieve the desired target cranial morphology and features (**Figure 3**). Most reported techniques are based on free-hand approaches requiring extensive manual human interaction, and the planning results are still highly dependent on the physicians' experience [41, 42].

Automatic surgical planning methodologies have been developed to find a personalized and optimal shape to target during the intervention [20]. Porras et al. [20] developed the first fully automatic and objective framework for interventional planning of metopic craniosynostosis. First, the algorithm uses a statistical shape model generated from a set of healthy subjects to determine the closest normal cranial shape to target during the surgical intervention. Then, a global registration approach is employed to arrange the fragments in the most appropriate configuration considering the interactions between bone fragments and avoiding overlaps. The optimal configuration of fragments is found by minimizing the degree of malformation and curvature discrepancies of the cranium. This framework was improved in a second study [43] to include bending of the fragments and to allow the users to define the desired number of fragments for interventional planning. They virtually planned 15 patients with metopic craniosynostosis, obtaining optimal target cranial shapes in all cases. The algorithm could also be adapted for the interventional planning of other types of craniosynostosis, although this is future work to be developed.

Automatic planning software enables to adjust bone fragments in the most optimal configuration to achieve normal morphology, reducing the cranial malformation of craniosynostosis patients. However, the results of longitudinal studies of the cranial growth of craniosynostosis patients indicate inadequate development following surgery [44]. Therefore, overcorrections considering growth and relapse must be factored into the surgical plan to ensure optimal long-term esthetic and functional outcomes [45]. Nowadays, there are no methodologies for automatic interventional planning of craniosynostosis integrating and considering overcorrection during the configuration of bone fragments. Future research is necessary to automatically determine the optimal degree of overcorrection for each patient, and to apply this overcorrection to the preoperative virtual surgical plan.

4. Computer-aided design and manufacturing

Transforming the preoperative virtual plan into a reality is a challenging endeavor and it is highly dependent on the surgical experience and judgment of the craniofacial surgeons. Computer-aided design and manufacturing (CAD/CAM) enables the fabrication of patient-specific cutting guides and shaping templates that can be used during surgery to guide osteotomy and remodeling according to the preoperative virtual plan [40].

Using a 3D reconstruction of the cranial surface as a reference, surgical cutting guides are designed to fit into the affected anatomical region (**Figure 4a**) and to guide the location of osteotomies as defined during the planning stage (**Figure 4b**) [12]. In addition, shaping templates can also be designed to assist during the intraoperative remodeling of the cranial vault [8, 46]. These templates enable the configuration of the resected bone fragments following the design decided during planning. Each of the fragments is fitted into their corresponding position on the template (**Figure 4c** and **d**) and rigidly fixed using resorbable plates and screws.

Accurate 3D reconstructions of the cranium are required to ensure optimal design and application of CAD/CAM guides and templates. CT imaging is the standard technique used for the generation of 3D models of the cranium prior to surgery. However, a new MRI technique called "black bone" has already been validated as a reference for CAD/CAM craniosynostosis surgery [47]. Therefore, MRI could be used to avoid CT scans and the exposure of the infants to ionizing radiation.

Fabrication of the patient-specific surgical cutting guides and templates must ensure a fast availability and secure sterilization without the risk of deformation. For this reason, manufacturing is commonly performed with selective laser sintering and polyamide material [12]. Other approaches have proposed the use

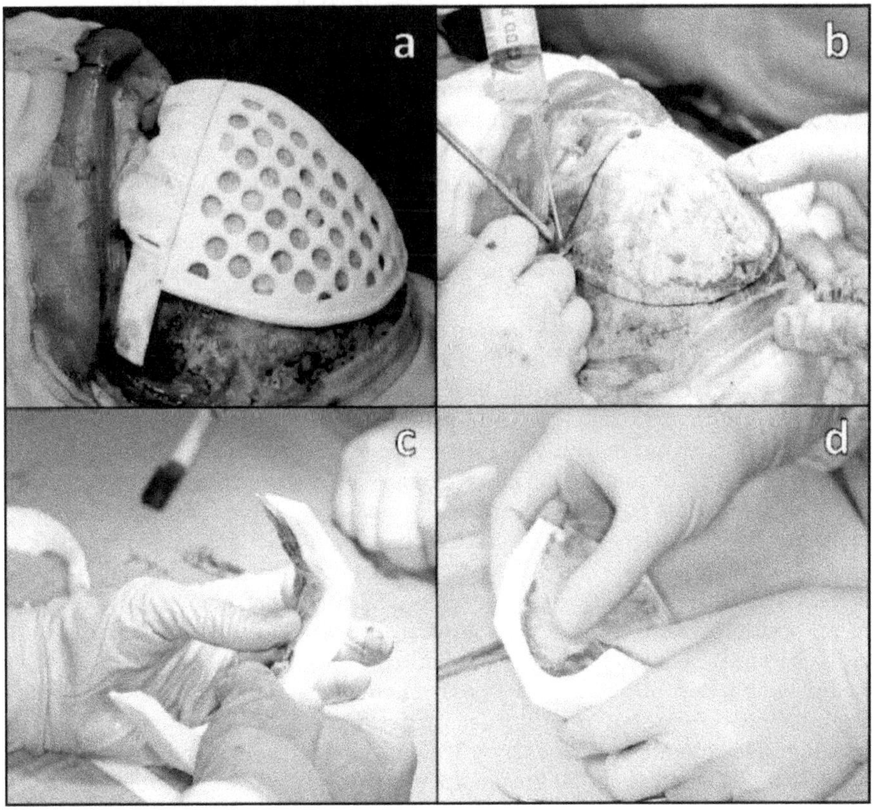

Figure 4.
Cutting guides and templates used during fronto-orbital advancement for surgical correction of a patient with metopic craniosynostosis. (a) Placement of surgical cutting guides on the calvarium, (b) marking of planned osteotomies on the calvarium, (c) shaping template for supraorbital bar remodeling, and (d) shaping template for frontal bone remodeling. Image adapted from [12].

of stainless steel templates [48]. Both types of materials can be sterilized before surgery using standard autoclave protocols [46].

Several studies have demonstrated the advantages of combining virtual surgical planning and CAD/CAM guides and templates for craniosynostosis surgery [8, 40, 45, 49]. This technology has been applied to single-suture and multiple-suture craniosynostosis [50]. Results indicate improved surgical outcomes and reduced operative time. Also, these technologies could reduce the experiential gap between younger and veteran craniofacial surgeons by accelerating the learning curve of future trainees. Overall, these studies demonstrate that the inclusion of this technology in the surgical workflow improves the efficiency, accuracy, and reproducibility of the interventions.

5. Image-guided surgery

The use of patient-specific CAD/CAM cutting guides and templates enables cutting the affected bone tissue and remodeling of the bone fragments as defined during the virtual surgical plan. However, after remodeling, reshaped bone tissue must be manually placed and fixed to the patient. In most cases, the placement of the reshaped bone tissue is assessed visually, and the final position may differ from the preoperative plan. Therefore, surgical outcomes can be compromised by slight positional and rotational variations of the remodeled bone tissue position.

In this context, different methodologies have been reported to assist during bone fragment placement. Hochfeld et al. [51] proposed the use of a stereotactic frame and Schanz screws to control the position of the fragments during the remodeling phase. Individual bone fragments are attached to the Schanz screws by bone brackets and configured based on a reference cranial shape obtained from a statistical shape model. Then, the frame is assembled in the surgical field to confirm fragment positions, and, finally, the remodeled fragments are rigidly fixed to each other by resorbable plates. Although the preliminary results obtained with this frame-based remodeling approach are positive, the incorporation of this technique into the standard clinical practice is limited by the increased surgical time, complexity, and invasiveness associated with the fixation of the frame to the patient.

Later on, Kobets et al. [52] described a guidance system to confirm bone fragment placement through the use of intraoperative CT imaging. First, remodeling of the cranial vault is performed exclusively based on the subjective assessment of the surgeons. Then, an intraoperative CT imaging scan is acquired and aligned with the preoperative plan for comparison and analysis. Finally, any necessary corrections in the bone fragment positions are applied before surgery is completed. Although intraoperative CT imaging provides accurate 3D reconstructions of the patient's anatomy, this technique requires the exposure of the infant to ionizing radiation, increases operative time, and does not enable real-time adjustment of bone fragments position to achieve the desired surgical outcome. Therefore, its application into the standard clinical practice is also limited.

In this situation, 3D photography has been suggested for intraoperative imaging and guidance during craniosynostosis surgery (**Figure 5**) [53]. In contrast to CT imaging, 3D photography can generate 3D models of the patient's anatomy without harmful ionizing radiation. This technology has already been successfully applied for diagnosis [34] and evaluation of surgical outcomes in craniosynostosis [36]. The mobility of hand-held 3D photography devices enables their use inside the operating room for intraoperative quantification. During the scanning process, the mobile device can be moved around the surgical field to acquire 3D models of the cranial vault during open cranial vault remodeling. Acquired intraoperative 3D

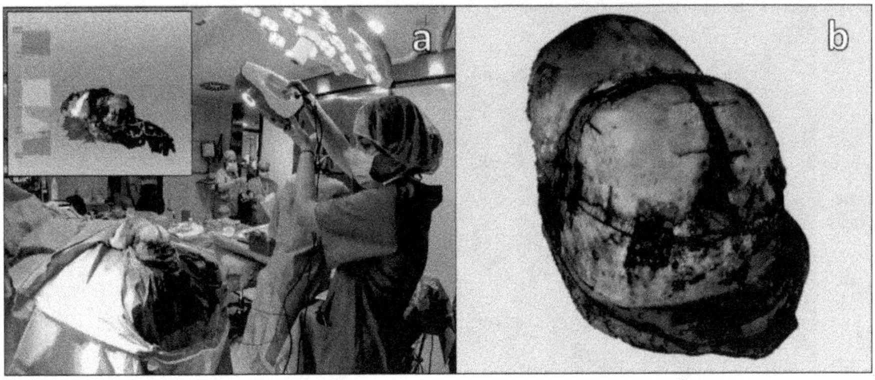

Figure 5.
(a) Acquisition of an intraoperative 3D photograph of the cranial vault during craniosynostosis surgery using the hand-held structured light scanner. (b) Acquired 3D photograph of the remodeled cranial vault.

photographs can be aligned with the preoperative virtual surgical plan for comparison and analysis (**Figure 6**) [54]. Overlaying of the actual and planned outcomes allows studying the accuracy of the surgical intervention and defining any necessary corrections to improve the outcome. This innocuous scanning technique can be used to acquire multiple scans during surgery to provide guidance to surgeons and to ensure optimal surgical outcomes.

Previously mentioned methodologies based on intraoperative CT imaging [52] or 3D photography [53] do not provide real-time feedback to the surgeons. Although multiple CT scans or 3D photographs could be acquired during surgery for more accurate and continuous guidance, this methodology would be limited by the increased operative time and, in the case of CT imaging, by the increased exposure to ionizing radiation.

An intraoperative navigation system has been specifically developed for real-time guidance during craniosynostosis reconstructions surgeries [12]. This system tracks the position of a surgical tool, which can then record points along the surface of the remodeled bone tissue. Then, the recorded position of the fragments can be compared with the target position defined during the planning phase, providing accurate and iterative quantitative feedback to surgeons (**Figure 7**). Navigation can

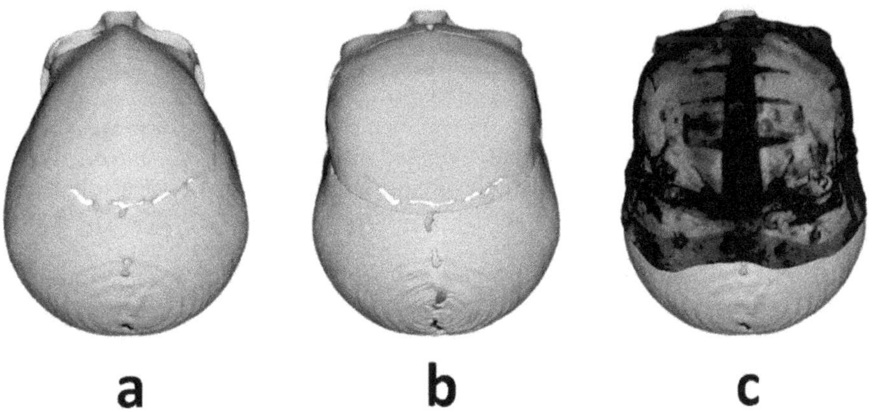

Figure 6.
Superior view of (a) preoperative model obtained from CT scan, (b) virtual surgical plan, and (c) intraoperative 3D photograph after cranial vault remodeling. Adapted from [12].

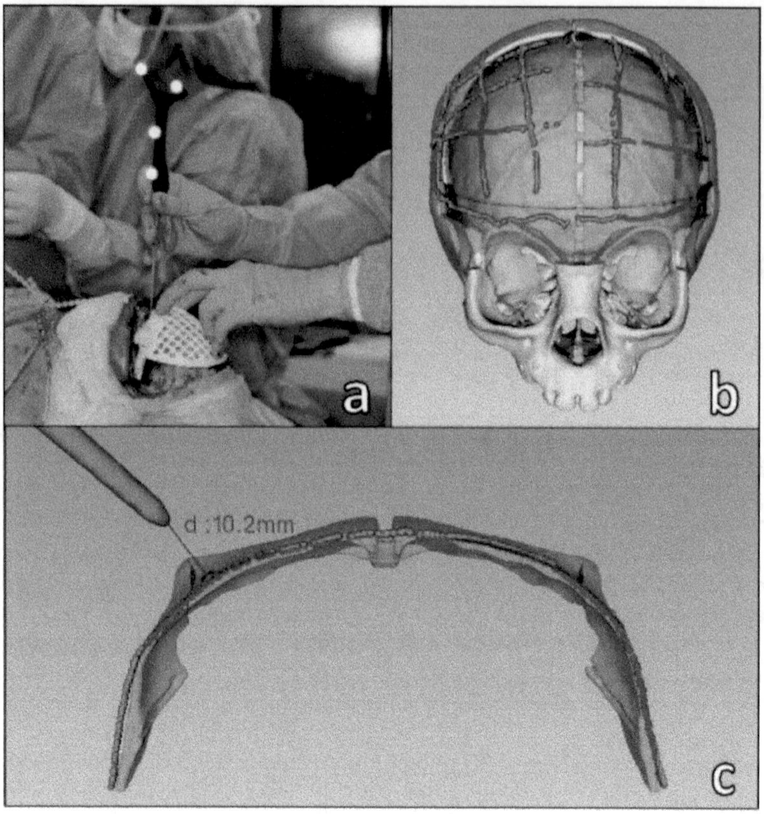

Figure 7.
Intraoperative navigation system: (a) surgeon recording registration points using tracked pointer tool; (b) points recorded by the navigation systems on the remodeled bone surface (red) and virtual surgical planning (green); (c) navigation of supraorbital bar region using tracked pointer tool. Image adapted from [12].

be used multiple times during surgery, making any necessary correction to ensure accurate matching with the preoperative virtual plan. This system has already been tested in five patients suffering from single-suture craniosynostosis in combination with CAD/CAM cutting guides and templates. The results of the study indicate high navigation accuracy (< 1 mm) and optimal surgical outcomes.

Although intraoperative navigation has demonstrated high accuracy and feasible integration into the surgical workflow, it presents some potential limitations. First, it requires the use of an optical tracking system in the operating room to track the position of the bone fragments. This hardware increases the cost associated with craniosynostosis surgery and may not be available in all centers for clinical deployment. Secondly, the navigation information is displayed on an external screen adjacent to the surgical field. Therefore, surgeons need to look at two different information sources and then mentally match the virtual data from the screen with the patient's anatomy. This visualization technique increases their cognitive load and may affect hand-eye coordination during the procedure.

Augmented reality (AR) technology has been applied in the medical field and, more specifically, to surgical procedures. AR enables the surgeons to focus on the surgical field while having access to external virtual information which is overlaid on the scene. This technology has already demonstrated to improve the accuracy and safety of surgical procedures [55].

Han et al. [56] reported the use of AR technology for guidance during open cranial vault reconstructions for the correction of craniosynostosis. Their methodology is based on the attachment of AR markers using occlusal splints for the alignment of virtual models in the AR visualization. An external high-definition camera captures images of the surgical field, which are then augmented and displayed to the surgeons on an external screen. The system was successfully tested on seven patients presenting plagiocephaly, but without evaluating the accuracy of AR. However, a thorough characterization of the accuracy of AR guidance is required before its clinical deployment.

Another work has proposed an AR visualization system for navigation of craniosynostosis surgeries [57]. It uses structured light scanning and sterilizable AR markers attached to the bone surface to ensure accurate alignment of the virtual models in the AR visualization. This methodology presents a significant improvement with respect to previous approaches [56], since the AR markers can be located using structured light scanning and attached near the region of interest to minimize alignment error. This system enables the visualization of the virtual plan overlaid on the surgical field, indicating the planes for bone osteotomy and the target position of remodeled bone fragments (**Figure 8**). The performance of the system has been evaluated on several 3D printed phantoms, obtaining a submillimetric accuracy when guiding both osteotomy and remodeling phases of the intervention. Moreover, the system has been successfully tested in two patients demonstrating the feasibility for integration in the surgical workflow and obtaining positive feedback from craniofacial surgeons. The AR visualization software is compatible with external cameras, smartphones, and head-mounted displays and, therefore, surgeons can choose the desired visualization platform according to their preferences and surgical needs. The main limitation of this system is that poor lighting conditions or occlusions of the markers may interrupt tracking and even cause inaccuracies in the AR display. However, illumination of the surgical field during interventions is usually homogeneous, and the position of the markers can be defined to avoid occlusions and maximize tracking capabilities.

While intraoperative navigation is a well-established technique for guidance in craniofacial surgery, AR visualization has recently emerged in the medical

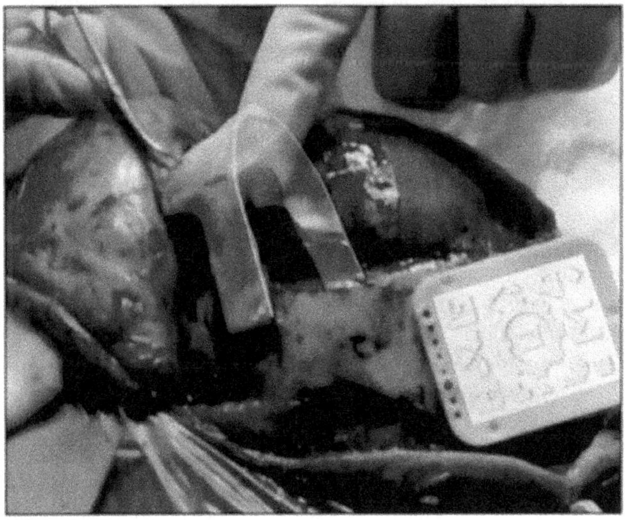

Figure 8.
Visualization of virtual surgical planning (green) overlaid on the surgical field during craniosynostosis surgery.

field and has not been yet integrated into the standard of care. Navigation systems are characterized by their accuracy and robustness during surgical instrument tracking with respect to patient anatomy [58]. On the other hand, AR technology is still under development and future research is still required to achieve optimal performance and robustness. Intraoperative guidance could benefit from the mixed integration of both technologies in the operating room to combine real-time and accurate positioning feedback provided by navigation systems with valuable AR visualization within the surgical field. Although both technologies require specialized training of craniofacial surgeons, proficiency could be achieved by the trainees through simulation-based training using realistic phantoms [59].

6. Conclusions

Multiple technological developments have demonstrated a positive impact on the management of craniosynostosis, from the diagnosis to the postoperative patient follow-up. Cranial shape analysis based on statistical shape models contributes to a more objective and precise diagnosis of craniosynostosis that will lead to earlier detection and surgical correction. Furthermore, statistical shape models can improve preoperative planning by determining the most optimal cranial shapes to target during surgical interventions and facilitating the automatic virtual arrangement of bone fragments. This target cranial shape enables to evaluate the stability of the surgical outcome during postoperative cranial development and to identify possible relapses. In that manner, it will be possible to assess the need for overcorrection to compensate for cranial underdevelopment after surgical remodeling.

Also, the use of CAD/CAM tools, intraoperative navigation, and augmented reality will enable the accurate translation of the preoperative plan into the operating room to ensure optimal surgical outcomes. All these technologies can be integrated into the surgical workflow to increase reproducibility, to reduce operative time, to streamline the methodology, and to reduce intersurgeon variability in open cranial vault remodeling procedures.

In addition, it has been demonstrated that 3D photography presents a valuable alternative to CT imaging. This non-invasive scanning technology can be easily used for diagnosis, intraoperative surgical outcome evaluation, and patient follow-up of craniosynostosis patients avoiding the exposure of the infants to harmful ionizing radiation. Besides, 3D photographs can be acquired instantly, and sedation or anesthesia is not required.

Most of the technological developments presented in this chapter have been tested and validated in non-syndromic single-suture synostosis. However, these approaches could also be applied to syndromic multi-suture synostosis. In these complex cases, most anatomical references in the cranium are altered and optimal surgical correction is challenging. Therefore, these cases will highly benefit from computer-assisted diagnosis, planning, and intraoperative guidance to achieve optimal surgical outcomes. Furthermore, these techniques could also be applied to secondary surgical interventions performed to correct possible complications or relapses after initial treatment.

Although all technologies mentioned can greatly benefit the management of craniosynostosis, there are some limitations to bear in mind. First of all, most of these technologies are costly, and this factor may restrict their integration into clinical practice in some centers with limited budgets. However, many of the previously mentioned technological developments are based on free and open-source software platforms [12, 53], which could reduce the costs associated with its integration on the surgical workflow. Also, CAD/CAM guides and templates can be designed and manufactured in-hospital to reduce cost and production time [60, 61]. These technologies could also be shared among different hospital departments, improving their impact at a lower cost.

Apart from the economic perspective, some indirect costs must also be considered. The addition of advanced cranial shape analysis, automatic planning algorithms, and design and manufacturing of CAD/CAM tools may increase the duration of the planning phase and will also require the collaboration of engineers. However, patient-specific planning of craniosynostosis surgeries is essential to improve surgical treatment. Advanced algorithms can provide valuable objective metrics to determine the best remodeling approach for each patient. Therefore, the benefits of these technological advancements may outweigh the increased duration of the preoperative planning phase.

In addition, most of the technologies developed for image-guided craniosynostosis surgeries require specialized training for craniofacial surgeons and some of them present a steep learning curve. However, surgeries can be simulated preoperatively using patient-specific phantoms to provide the trainees with realistic tactile feedback of the patient's anatomy. Simulation offers a safe environment where surgery can be replicated step-by-step leading to the acquisition of technical skills which can be translated into better performance during the surgical task [59].

To conclude, multiple technologies are currently available to improve the surgical management of craniosynostosis. The integration of these developments on the surgical workflow of craniosynostosis will have a positive impact on the surgical outcomes, increasing the reproducibility and efficiency of these procedures. Multidisciplinary collaborations between scientific and clinical personnel are essential to improve patient care. Further studies must evaluate the cost-effectiveness of these technologies to determine how to integrate them optimally into clinical practice.

Acknowledgements

Supported by projects PI18/01625 (Ministerio de Ciencia, Innovación y Universidades, Instituto de Salud Carlos III and European Regional Development Fund "Una manera de hacer Europa") and IND2018/TIC-9753 (Comunidad de Madrid).

Conflict of interest

The authors declare that they have no conflicts of interest.

Author details

David García-Mato[1,2], Javier Pascau[1,2]* and Santiago Ochandiano[2,3]

1 Department of Bioengineering and Aerospace Engineering, Universidad Carlos III de Madrid, Madrid, Spain

2 Gregorio Marañón Health Research Institute, Madrid, Spain

3 Department of Oral and Maxillofacial Surgery, Hospital General Universitario Gregorio Marañón, Madrid, Spain

*Address all correspondence to: jpascau@ing.uc3m.es

References

[1] Sharma R. Craniosynostosis. Indian J Plast Surg. 2013;46(1):18.

[2] Cohen SR, Frank RC, Meltzer HS, Levy ML. Craniosynostosis. Handb Craniomaxillofacial Surg. 2014;343-68.

[3] Boulet SL, Rasmussen SA, Honein MA. A population-based study of craniosynostosis in metropolitan Atlanta, 1989-2003. Am J Med Genet Part A. 2008;146(8):984-91.

[4] Kweldam CF, Van Der Vlugt JJ, Van Der Meulen JJNM. The incidence of craniosynostosis in the Netherlands, 1997-2007. J Plast Reconstr Aesthetic Surg [Internet]. 2011;64(5):583-8. Available from: http://dx.doi.org/10.1016/j.bjps.2010.08.026

[5] Jimenez DF, Barone CM. Early treatment of anterior calvarial craniosynostosis using endoscopic-assisted minimally invasive techniques. 2007;1411-9.

[6] Cohen SR, Holmes RE, Ozgur BM, Meltzer HS, Levy ML. Fronto-orbital and cranial osteotomies with resorbable fixation using an endoscopic approach. Clin Plast Surg. 2004 Jul;31(3):429-42, vi.

[7] Persing JA. MOC-PS(SM) CME Article: Management Considerations in the Treatment of Craniosynostosis. Plast Reconstr Surg. 2008;121(Supplement):1-11.

[8] Mardini S, Alsubaie S, Cayci C, Chim H, Wetjen N. Three-dimensional preoperative virtual planning and template use for surgical correction of craniosynostosis. J Plast Reconstr Aesthetic Surg. 2014;67(3):336-43.

[9] Slater BJ, Lenton KA, Kwan MD, Gupta DM, Wan DC, Longaker MT. Cranial sutures: A brief review. Plast Reconstr Surg. 2008;121(4):170-8.

[10] Hirabayashi S, Sugawara Y, Sakurai A, Harii K. Frontoorbital advancement by gradual distraction. J Neurosurg. 1998;89(6):1058-61.

[11] Gomi A, Sunaga A, Kamochi H, Oguma H, Sugawara Y. Distraction osteogenesis update: Introduction of multidirectional cranial distraction osteogenesis. J Korean Neurosurg Soc. 2016;59(3):233-41.

[12] García-Mato D, Ochandiano S, García-Sevilla M, Navarro-Cuéllar C, Darriba-Allés J V, García-Leal R, et al. Craniosynostosis surgery: workflow based on virtual surgical planning, intraoperative navigation and 3D printed patient-specific guides and templates. Sci Rep. 2019;9(1):17691.

[13] Whitaker LA, Bartlett SP, Schut L, Bruce D. Craniosynostosis: an analysis of the timing, treatment, and complications in 164 consecutive patients. Plast Reconstr Surg [Internet]. 1987 Aug [cited 2018 Aug 28];80(2):195-212. Available from: http://www.ncbi.nlm.nih.gov/pubmed/3602170

[14] McCarthy JG., Glasberg SB., Cutting CB., Epstein FJ., Grayson BH., Ruff G., et al. Twenty-year experience with early surgery for craniosynostosis: I. Isolated craniofacial synostosis--results and unsolved problems. Plast Reconstr Surg. 1995;96(2):272-83.

[15] Greenberg BM, Schneider SJ. Trigonocephaly: surgical considerations and long term evaluation. J Craniofac Surg. 2006 May;17(3):528-35.

[16] Selber JC, Brooks C, Kurichi JE, Temmen T, Sonnad SS, Whitaker LA. Long-term results following fronto-orbital reconstruction in nonsyndromic unicoronal synostosis. Plast Reconstr Surg. 2008;121(5):251-60.

[17] Pearson GD, Havlik RJ, Eppley B, Nykiel M, Sadove AM. Craniosynostosis:

a single institution's outcome assessment from surgical reconstruction. J Craniofac Surg. 2008 Jan;19(1):65-71.

[18] Seruya M, Oh AK, Boyajian MJ, Posnick JC, Myseros JS, Yaun AL, et al. Long-term outcomes of primary craniofacial reconstruction for craniosynostosis: A 12-year experience. Plast Reconstr Surg. 2011;127(6): 2397-406.

[19] Engel M, Castrillon-Oberndorfer G, Hoffmann J, Mühling J, Seeberger R, Freudlsperger C. Long-term results in nonsyndromatic unilateral coronal synostosis treated with fronto-orbital advancement. J Craniomaxillofac Surg. 2013 Dec;41(8):747-54.

[20] Porras AR, Zukic D, Equobahrie A, Rogers GF, Linguraru MG. Personalized Optimal Planning for the Surgical Correction of Metopic Craniosynostosis. Clin image-based Proced from Plan to Interv Int Work CLIP ., held conjunction with MICCAI . Revis Sel Pap CLIP. 2016;2016:60-7.

[21] Steinbacher DM. Three-Dimensional Analysis and Surgical Planning in Craniomaxillofacial Surgery. J Oral Maxillofac Surg. 2015;73(12):S40-56.

[22] Saber NR, Phillips J, Looi T, Usmani Z, Burge J, Drake J, et al. Generation of normative pediatric skull models for use in cranial vault remodeling procedures. Child's Nerv Syst. 2012;28(3):405-10.

[23] Mendoza CS, Safdar N, Okada K, Myers E, Rogers GF, Linguraru MG. Personalized assessment of craniosynostosis via statistical shape modeling. Med Image Anal. 2014;18(4):635-46.

[24] Kotrikova B, Krempien R, Freier K, Mühling J. Diagnostic imaging in the management of craniosynostoses. Eur Radiol [Internet]. 2007;17(8):1968-78. Available from: https://doi.org/10.1007/s00330-006-0520-y

[25] Marcus JR, Domeshek LF, Loyd AM, Schoenleber JM, Das RR, Nightingale RW, et al. Use of a three-dimensional, normative database of pediatric craniofacial morphology for modern anthropometric analysis. Plast Reconstr Surg. 2009;124(6):2076-84.

[26] Dean D, Bookstein FL, Koneru S, Lee JH, Kamath J, Cutting CB, et al. Average African American three-dimensional computed tomography skull images: The potential clinical importance of ethnicity and sex. Vol. 9, Journal of Craniofacial Surgery. 1998. p. 348-59.

[27] Mendoza CS, Safdar N, Myers E, Kittisarapong T, Rogers GF, Linguraru MG. An optimal set of landmarks for metopic craniosynostosis diagnosis from shape analysis of pediatric CT scans of the head. Med Imaging 2013 Comput Diagnosis. 2013;8670:86702T.

[28] Wood BC, Mendoza CS, Oh AK, Myers E, Safdar N, Linguraru MG, et al. What's in a Name? Accurately Diagnosing Metopic Craniosynostosis Using a Computational Approach. Plast Reconstr Surg. 2015;137(1):205-13.

[29] Robertson E, Kwan P, Louie G, Boulanger P, Aalto D. Test-retest validation of a cranial deformity index in unilateral coronal craniosynostosis. Comput Methods Biomech Biomed Engin [Internet]. 2020;0(0):1-13. Available from: https://doi.org/10.1080/10255842.2020.1795143

[30] Tenhagen M, Bruse JL, Rodriguez-florez N, Angullia F, Borghi A, Koudstaal MJ, et al. Three-Dimensional Handheld Scanning to Quantify Head-Shape Changes in Spring-Assisted Surgery for Sagittal Craniosynostosis. J Craniofac Surg. 2016;27(8):2117-23.

[31] Branson HM, Shroff MM. Craniosynostosis and 3-Dimensional Computed Tomography. Semin

Ultrasound, CT MRI [Internet]. 2011;32(6):569-77. Available from: http://www.sciencedirect.com/science/article/pii/S0887217111000989

[32] Schweitzer T, Böhm H, Meyer-Marcotty P, Collmann H, Ernestus RI, Krauß J. Avoiding CT scans in children with single-suture craniosynostosis. Child's Nerv Syst. 2012;28(7):1077-82.

[33] Wong JY, Oh AK, Ohta E, Hunt AT, Rogers GF, Mulliken JB, et al. Validity and reliability of craniofacial anthropometric measurement of 3D digital photogrammetric images. Cleft Palate-Craniofacial J. 2008;45(3):232-9.

[34] Meulstee JW, Verhamme LM, Borstlap WA, Van der Heijden F, De Jong GA, Xi T, et al. A new method for three-dimensional evaluation of the cranial shape and the automatic identification of craniosynostosis using 3D stereophotogrammetry. Int J Oral Maxillofac Surg. 2017;46(7):819-26.

[35] Wilbrand JF, Szczukowski A, Blecher JC, Pons-Kuehnemann J, Christophis P, Howaldt HP, et al. Objectification of cranial vault correction for craniosynostosis by three-dimensional photography. J Cranio-Maxillofacial Surg [Internet]. 2012;40(8):726-30. Available from: http://dx.doi.org/10.1016/j.jcms.2012.01.007

[36] Porras AR, Tu L, Tsering D, Mantilla E, Oh A, Enquobahrie A, et al. Quantification of head shape from three-dimensional photography for pre- and post-surgical evaluation of craniosynostosis. Plast Reconstr Surg [Internet]. 2019 Aug; Available from: https://doi.org/10.1097/PRS.0000000000006260

[37] Freudlsperger C, Steinmacher S, Bächli H, Somlo E, Hoffmann J, Engel M. Metopic synostosis: Measuring intracranial volume change following fronto-orbital advancement using three-dimensional photogrammetry. J Cranio-Maxillofacial Surg [Internet]. 2015;43(5):593-8. Available from: http://www.sciencedirect.com/science/article/pii/S1010518215000487

[38] Rodriguez-Florez N, Göktekin ÖK, Bruse JL, Borghi A, Angullia F, Knoops PGM, et al. Quantifying the effect of corrective surgery for trigonocephaly: A non-invasive, non-ionizing method using three-dimensional handheld scanning and statistical shape modelling. J Cranio-Maxillofacial Surg [Internet]. 2017;45(3):387-94. Available from: http://www.sciencedirect.com/science/article/pii/S1010518217300021

[39] Kirmi O, Lo SJ, Johnson D, Anslow P. Craniosynostosis: A Radiological and Surgical Perspective. Semin Ultrasound, CT MRI. 2009;30(6):492-512.

[40] Seruya M, Borsuk DE, Khalifian S, Carson BS, Dalesio NM, Dorafshar AH. Computer-Aided Design and Manufacturing in Craniosynostosis Surgery. J Craniofac Surg. 2013;24(4):1100-5.

[41] Havlik RJ, Azurin DJ, Bartlett SP, Whitaker LA. Analysis and treatment of severe trigonocephaly. Plast Reconstr Surg. 1999 Feb;103(2):381-90.

[42] Selber J, Reid RR, Gershman B, Sonnad SS, Sutton LN, Whitaker LA, et al. Evolution of Operative Techniques for the Treatment of Single-Suture Metopic Synostosis. Ann Plast Surg [Internet]. 2007;59(1). Available from: https://journals.lww.com/annalsplasticsurgery/Fulltext/2007/07000/Evolution_of_Operative_Techniques_for_the.2.aspx

[43] Porras AR, Paniagua B, Ensel S, Keating R, Rogers GF, Enquobahrie A, et al. Locally Affine Diffeomorphic Surface Registration and Its Application to Surgical Planning of Fronto-Orbital Advancement. IEEE Trans Med Imaging. 2018;37(7):1690-700.

[44] Fearon JA, Ditthakasem K, Chan WNJ, Herbert M. Long-Term Growth following Trigonocephaly Repairs: Are Overcorrections Necessary? Plast Reconstr Surg [Internet]. 2020;145(3). Available from: https://journals.lww.com/plasreconsurg/Fulltext/2020/03000/Long_Term_Growth_following_Trigonocephaly_Repairs_.33.aspx

[45] Khechoyan DY, Saber NR, Burge J, Fattah A, Drake J, Forrest CR, et al. Surgical outcomes in craniosynostosis reconstruction: The use of prefabricated templates in cranial vault remodelling. J Plast Reconstr Aesthetic Surg. 2014;67(1):9-16.

[46] Soleman J, Thieringer F, Beinemann J, Kunz C, Guzman R. Computer-assisted virtual planning and surgical template fabrication for frontoorbital advancement. 2015;38(May):1-8.

[47] Lethaus B, Gruichev D, Gräfe D, Bartella AK, Hahnel S, Yovev T, et al. "Black bone": the new backbone in CAD/CAM-assisted craniosynostosis surgery? Acta Neurochir (Wien) [Internet]. 2020; Available from: https://doi.org/10.1007/s00701-020-04445-z

[48] Burge J, Saber NR, Looi T, French B, Usmani Z, Anooshiravani N, et al. Application of CAD/CAM Prefabricated Age-Matched Templates in Cranio-Orbital Remodeling in Craniosynostosis. J Craniofac Surg. 2011;22(5):1810-3.

[49] Queiros C, Joly A, Paré A, Listrat A, Travers N, Goga D, et al. Use of cutting guides during craniosynostosis sequelae surgery: A comparative study between computer-assisted planning and post-operative results. J Cranio-Maxillofacial Surg. 2017;45(7):1062-8.

[50] Iyer RR, Wu A, Macmillan A, Musavi L, Cho R, Lopez J, et al. Use of computer-assisted design and manufacturing to localize dural venous sinuses during reconstructive surgery for craniosynostosis. Childs Nerv Syst. 2018 Jan;34(1):137-42.

[51] Hochfeld M, Lamecker H, Thomale U-W, Schulz M, Zachow S, Haberl H. Frame-based cranial reconstruction. J Neurosurg Pediatr. 2014;13(3):319-23.

[52] Kobets AJ, Ammar A, Nakhla J, Scoco A, Nasser R, Goodrich JT, et al. Virtual modeling, stereolithography, and intraoperative CT guidance for the optimization of sagittal synostosis reconstruction: a technical note. Child's Nerv Syst. 2018;34(5):965-70.

[53] García-Mato D, García-Sevilla M, Ochandiando S, Navarro-Cuéllar C, Darriba-Allés JV, García-Leal R, et al. Structured Light Scanning for Morphometric Analysis in Craniosynostosis Reconstruction Surgery. In: International Journal of Computer Assisted Radiology and Surgery. Rennes, France; 2019. p. 40-1.

[54] García-Mato D, García-Sevilla M, Ochandiando S, Moreta-Martinez R, Darriba-Allés JV, García-Leal R, et al. Intraoperative Outcome Evaluation in Craniosynostosis Reconstruction Surgery using 3D Photography. In: International Journal of Computer Assisted Radiology and Surgery. Munich, Germany; 2020. p. 87-8.

[55] Berryman DR. Augmented Reality: A Review. Med Ref Serv Q. 2012;31(2):212-8.

[56] Han W, Yang X, Wu S, Fan S, Chen X, Aung ZM, et al. A new method for cranial vault reconstruction: Augmented reality in synostotic plagiocephaly surgery. J Cranio-Maxillofacial Surg. 2019;47(8):1280-4.

[57] García-Mato D, Moreta-Martinez R, García-Sevilla M, Ochandiano S, García-Leal R, Pérez-Mañanes R, et al. Augmented Reality Visualization for Craniosynostosis Surgery. Comput Methods Biomech Biomed Eng Imaging Vis. 2020;

[58] Peters T, Cleary K. Image-guided interventions: Technology and applications. Image-Guided Interventions: Technology and Applications. 2008. 1-557 p.

[59] Palter VN, Grantcharov TP. Simulation in surgical education. Can Med Assoc J [Internet]. 2010 Aug 10;182(11):1191 LP – 1196. Available from: http://www.cmaj.ca/content/182/11/1191.abstract

[60] Arnal-Burró J, Pérez-Mañanes R, Gallo-del-Valle E, Igualada-Blazquez C, Cuervas-Mons M, Vaquero-Martín J. Three dimensional-printed patient-specific cutting guides for femoral varization osteotomy: Do it yourself. Knee [Internet]. 2017 Dec 1;24(6):1359-68. Available from: https://doi.org/10.1016/j.knee.2017.04.016

[61] Moreta-Martinez R, García-Mato D, García-Sevilla M, Pérez-Mañanes R, Calvo-Haro J, Pascau J. Augmented reality in computer-assisted interventions based on patient-specific 3D printed reference. Healthc Technol Lett. 2018;5(5):162-6.

Chapter 7

Craniofacial Corrective Surgery in Syndromic Craniosynostosis

Khairul Bariah Chi Adam, Firdaus Hariri, Wei Lee Chee, Kathiravan Purmal, Mohd Faizal Abdullah and Nazer Berahim

Abstract

This surgical field has now progressed and becoming an established subspecialty involving various surgical disciplines worldwide. Various complex CMF syndromes reported in syndromic craniosynostosis include Crouzon, Apert and Pfeiffer syndromes. These syndromes carry specific functional discrepancies associated with the affected structural anomaly and may therefore have functional issues involving the brain, eye and airway among others. As corrective surgery is often indicated depending on the affected vital functions, other factors that need to be considered are patient's age, comorbidities, urgency, available expertise and patient's overall prognosis based on the degree of anomaly. As such, the corrective surgery can be categorized into; (1) intermediate which is performed at an early phase and aimed to improve or salvage important vital functions such as the brain, eye, airway or feeding which are important for the child's development and, (2) definitive treatment aimed at permanently correct the functional discrepancies. Intermediate corrective surgery may include invasive procedures such as ventriculo-peritoneal (VP) shunts, tarsorrhaphy, adenotonsillectomy and tracheostomy whereas definitive corrective surgery may include surgical procedures such as monobloc, Le Fort III osteotomy, posterior cranial vault expansion and mandibular advancement. This chapter will elaborate on the indications, types, challenges in the management and the proposed prevention measures in corrective surgery for specifically for syndromic craniosynostosis patients.

Keywords: corrective surgery, syndromic craniosynostosis, craniofacial surgery

1. Introduction

Syndromic craniosynostosis is a condition which involves premature fusion of multiple skull sutures and may be associated with extracranial deformities such as limb, cardiac and tracheal malformations [1, 2]. Therefore, this syndrome usually comes with related issues such as increased intracranial pressure which can cause visual impairment (increased intraocular pressure), sleep impairment and eating difficulties due to midface hypoplasia, and even risk of impairment of mental development [3]. There are about 150 syndromes associated with craniosynostosis namely Crouzon, Pfeiffer and Apert syndrome.

IntechOpen

Therefore, corrective surgery in syndromic craniosynostosis were developed in relation to its deformities and functional issues. Conventional craniofacial surgical techniques, such as strip craniectomy, fronto-orbital advancement, and Le Fort III procedures proved to be reliable to treat symptomatic syndromic craniosynostosis. However, limitations were observed in severe conditions where large segmental advancement were required, difficulty to close the gap primarily as well as inadequate stability secondary to soft tissue restriction and unstable bone segment fixation. These limitations thus causing relapse and creating less than an ideal long-term outcome [4]. Hence distraction osteogenesis (DO) were introduced to provide a reliable surgical alternative in achieving superior segmental advancement compared with conventional techniques in treating functional issues in syndromic craniosynostosis.

Syndromic craniosynostosis patients usually presented with multiple major functional disturbances which requires multi-disciplinary management including maxillofacial surgery, neurosurgery, plastic surgery and ENT among others. As such, the indication for each major surgery in paediatric patients with this condition should be discussed by the craniofacial team members as the procedure carries substantial mortality and morbidity risks [5].

2. Syndromic craniosynostosis and the genetic perspectives

Craniosynostosis was first known as craniostenosis that was introduced by German pathologist, Virchow in 1851. It was then changed to craniosynostosis and widely accepted ever since [6]. Craniosynostosis is a condition whereby the process of early or premature fusion of the skull sutures happens that leads to the unwanted growth pattern of the skull. The skull will not be able to grow perpendicular to the fused suture but instead will grow in parallel direction to the fused suture. The brain will use the space available to grow and cause an abnormal head shape and facial features [7]. In cases whereby the skull does not have any spaces due to fused sutures, the brain will continue to grow thus causing increased in intracranial pressure hence patient will develop visual disturbances, sleeping impairment due to airway disruption, eating difficulties because of unusual jaw growth and reduction in mental development.

Most known craniosynostosis cases are nonsyndromic and can occur as an isolated event or associated with other skeletal and developmental anomalies in specific clinical features for recognized syndromes. Patients who have been diagnosed with syndromic craniosynostosis are much more complex and require a multidisciplinary approach to effectively manage all the problems faced. Most of the syndromic craniosynostosis cases are due to genetic defect that may present as autosomal dominant, autosomal recessive and X-linked patterns of inheritance. The molecular genetic protocol for the diagnosis of syndromic craniosynostosis such Crouzon syndrome includes first-line tests of FGFR2 exons IgIIIa and IgIIIc followed by second-line tests of FGFR2 exons 3, 5, 11, and 14 to 17 and FGFR3 Pro250Arg and Ala391Glu as proposed by Wilkie et al. [7]. There are multiple types of syndromic craniosynostosis cases but almost all of the them shared the same craniomaxillofacial features such as exophthalmos, midface hypoplasia, cranial base anomalies as well as abnormal face with the additional limb anomalies [8–9]. Syndromic craniosynostosis occurs in 1:8750 newborns [10–13]. The most common syndromic craniosynostosis cases identified and managed are Crouzon, Apert, and Pfeiffer syndromes. These syndromes may be presented with identical craniomaxillofacial features. Therefore, it is prudent to differentiate to achieve an accurate diagnosis by relating to other features such digital or limb anomalies.

2.1 Crouzon syndromes

Clinically, patients may present with brachycephaly, small or shallow orbits with exophthalmos, midface hypoplasia and occlusal anterior open bite. However, there are no recorded cases that anomalies involving limbs are present. It is an autosomal dominant inheritance pattern that showed mutations in the fibroblast growth factor receptor 2 (FGFR-2) and occurred in 1 in 25,000 live births thus the most common syndromic craniosynostosis identified. Patients who have been diagnosed often have normal intelligence. Several cases identified as higher risk of increased intracranial pressure compared to other syndromic craniosynostosis cases [8, 14, 15]. The most common synostosis pattern observed is bicoronal synostosis which leads to brachycephalic shape, others such as scaphocephaly, trigonocephaly and cloverleaf skull have been diagnosed. Early fusion of cranial sutures resulted in shallow orbits and eye proptosis, small & high arched palate and anterior open bite. Eye proptosis or exorbitism can cause exposure conjunctivitis, keratitis, visual acuity problems and herniation of the globe. The synostosis will lead to midface hypoplasia as well and with normal development of mandible, class III skeletal profile & malocclusion formed. There are also other conditions reported such conductive hearing deficit, strabismus and hydrocephalus.

2.2 Apert syndromes

Often patients will present with turribrachycephaly, midface hypoplasia, symmetrical syndactyly of both hands and feet. It is also an autosomal dominant inheritance pattern with mutations in FGFR-2 occurring in 1 in 100,000 births with cases seen are sporadic new mutations. Bicoronal synostosis with large anterior fontanelle, bitemporal widening and occipital flattening is common presentation in most patients. In this syndrome, the midface hypoplasia is more severe than others with concavity of the face, very shallow orbits, mild hypertelorism and downslanting palpebral fissure, eye proptosis, cleft palate, anterior open bite. It will have the characteristic depressed nasal bridge and downward tip resulting in parrot beak deformity. The severe hypoplastic midface in Class III skeletal features will result in a small airway that causes airway compromise needing a tracheostomy to secure the airway.

Pathognomonic syndrome will be the hand syndactyly which often involve fusion of the second, third and fourth fingers that lead to middigital hand mass with the first and fifth fingers may also join. In certain cases, if the thumb is free, it is broad and deviates radially. In the feet, syndactyly will involve the second, third and fourth toes. Patients will suffer loss of function and referral to a hand surgeon is essential. Many patients have normal intelligence despite of some cases delayed mental development identified. Marruci et al. published the Great Ormond Street Hospital data on the expectant management of their patients in raised ICP in Apert syndrome. Their protocol is to offer cranial vault expansion only in the setting of confirmed elevation of ICP. Raised ICP developed in 83% of patients, 50% in the first year of life with the average age at onset was at 18 months. 35% of those treated successfully for their first episode however, went on to develop a second episode on average 3 years 4 months later [16].

2.3 Pfeiffer syndrome

Characterized by features of craniofacial anomalies from mild to severe condition. It includes turribrachycephaly, midface hypoplasia, exorbitism and the pathognomonic features of broad thumbs and great toes with variable soft tissue syndactyly. Other associated features include hypertelorism, strabismus, downslanting palpebral fissures, class III malocclusion and beaked nasal deformity. Again, the majority of cases involve FGFR-2 mutations, 5% of patients express an FGFR-1 mutation and demonstrate less severe phenotype [17, 18]. It is an autosomal dominant inheritance pattern with the incidence of 1 in 100,000 births. A classification system proposed that patients are categorized into three types based upon clinical findings and severity. Type 1 is the classic Pfeiffer syndrome clinical pattern. Type 2 is more severe and associated with the cloverleaf skull and type 3 Pfeiffer syndrome is the most severely affected. In one institution, a review of 28 patients has been conducted and the Cohen subtypes dissemination is 61% type 1, 25% type 2 and 14% type 3 [19]. All patients have undergone numerous corrective surgery. This study recommends aggressive treatment and monitoring on patients' functional conditions to prevent further damage to the vital organ that leads to permanent loss of function.

Therefore, syndromic craniosynostosis is a condition of multiple associated clinical problems with the same pattern of treatment strategies, expected difficulties and pathologic identifications. Profound knowledge of the disease process, pathognomonic findings and clinical situations of each syndrome is essential. Therefore, multidisciplinary approach in total management of the clinical problems is important and must be detected and treated earlier to improve patient's functional conditions and quality of life.

3. Corrective surgery

3.1 Pre-surgical assessment & preparation

In syndromic craniosynostosis, surgical intervention is often functionally indicated with the primary aim is to treat the pressing functional discrepancy or to salvage vital structures such as the brain and eyes [4, 20]. The three main functional issues secondary to the severe skull deformity are increased intracranial pressure, severe exopthalmos and obliterated nasopharyngeal airway. As such, comprehensive assessment to the brain, eyes and upper airway is paramount to determine the specific problem prior to any surgical decision.

3.1.1 Multi-disciplinary approach

Taking the multiple functional issues into consideration, multi-disciplinary approach has become the trend in syndromic craniosynostosis management. A craniofacial centre or unit may consist of various specialties such as neurosurgery, oral and maxillofacial surgery, plastic surgery, otorhinolaryngology, ophthalmology, and oculoplastic, among others.

3.1.2 General assessment

Patient growth progress and development should be assessed and properly documented as it provides valuable baseline and comparative data before and after surgery. This includes objective data such as head circumference, height, weight, gross and fine motor, as well as speech development, among others. These parameters are important as it may determine whether any corrective surgery should be indicated as early as possible or performed at a later stage [21].

3.1.3 Clinical assessment

Specifically on the craniofacial region, assessment can be focused on patient's initial head shape, the degree of exopthalmos, ability for eyelid closure, nasal airflow, midfacial projection, jaw relationship and intraoral condition. Clinical picture documentation is very useful as it can be used for serial comparison.

3.1.4 Imaging assessment

Imaging modalities provide valuable input in identifying a specific functional issue. Magnetic resonance imaging (MRI) or CT scan may indicate any anomaly in the brain region and the condition of skull bone, respectively. Thinning of bone or copper beaten appearance is an indication to raised intracranial pressure necessitating corrective surgery to improve the intracranial volume via procedures such as posterior vault expansion or fronto-orbital advancement as shown in **Figures 1** and **2**.

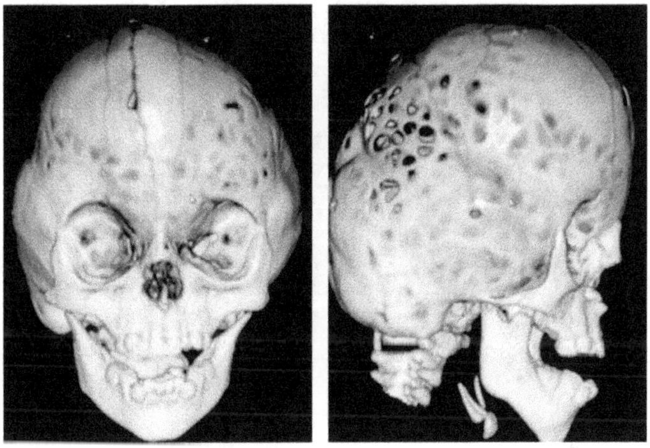

Figure 1.
Thinning of the skull bone noted from the reconstructed 3D CT scan.

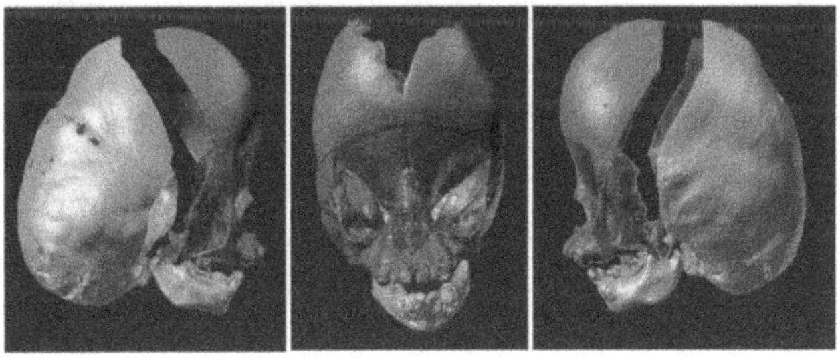

Figure 2.
Surgical simulation on the monobloc advancement of the frontofacial segment.

3.1.5 Ophthalmological assessment

Specific ophthalmological assessment such as retinal camera or fundoscopy provides information of the interior surface of the eye, including the retina, vasculature, optic disc and macula. Pale disc may be an indication of increased intracranial pressure. Tonometry can be performed to measure the intraocular pressure. Assessment of the volume of eye sockets is also important and can be conducted via the analysis of CT scan.

3.1.6 Airway assessment

For the airway, endoscopic examination is often performed to determine the cause of airway obliteration. The cause can either be due to soft tissue or hard tissue or both. Specific recognition of the anatomical restriction allows the surgical team to decide on the most ideal corrective surgical intervention such as shown in **Figure 3**. As most syndromic craniosynostosis patients are classically presented with midface hypoplasia, polysomnography (PSG) is the gold standard to diagnose obstructive sleep apnea (OSA).

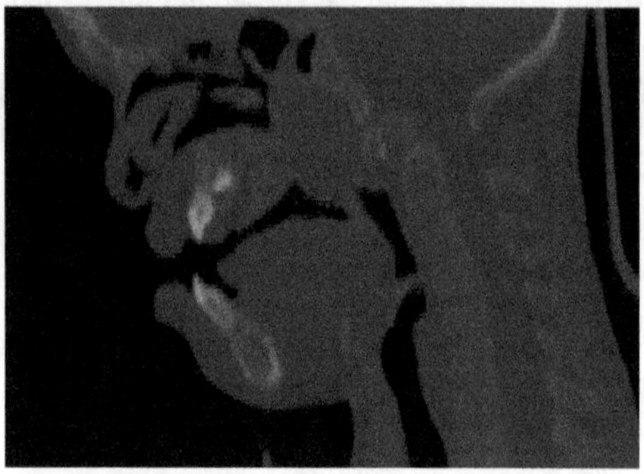

Figure 3.
Airway assessment using software and CT scan.

3.1.7 Pre-operative preparation

Other pre-surgical preparation includes patient optimization prior to surgery via comprehensive in ward assessment by paediatric respiratory physician and anaesthetist.

Patient's CT image can be used for surgical simulation using surgical software and utilized for 3D model fabrication to optimize the corrective surgery outcomes as shown in **Figure 4**. The technology provides precision and significantly reduces the operating hours thus minimizing the potential complication such as intra-operative bleeding [21–24]. All patients in the authors' center had their 3D skull bio-model fabricated to allow surgical simulation and vector determination to optimize the outcome of surgery. The pre-bending of the distractor footplates for the internal device and presurgical simulation proved critical because it contributed to the precision of device fixation and correct segmental movement to ensure a favorable final outcome and decrease operating time.

The selection of devices is based on device suitability and functional indications. Increased ICP was assessed by history, presence of signs or symptoms, imaging analysis, and ophthalmologic assessment. For the eye, the patients' ability to achieve eyelid closure was assessed and documented and supplemented with eye examinations that included optic disc condition and cup-to-disc ratio through funduscopy. Airway function was assessed by polysomnography and digital airway assessment.

Intra-operative complications should be anticipated thus preparation should include paediatric intensive care unit booking, blood cross-matched and reserve for transfusion as well as appropriate drug prescription.

When certain corrective surgery has been agreed by the multi-disciplinary team, consent should be clear and comprehensive with consideration of various complications ranging from mild to severe degree, at intra-operative and post-operative phase.

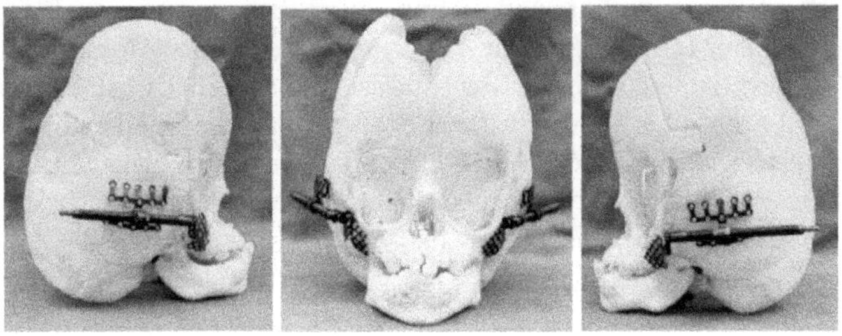

Figure 4.
Simulation of the surgical procedures using reconstructed 3D STL model from the CT scan.

3.2 Surgical techniques and its application

Following comprehensive assessment from the craniofacial team, the choice of surgery basically depends on the aim, condition of the patient, skill of the surgeons and the facility. Hariri et al. [25] proposed for a protocol to indicate the type of intervention based on the aim of the functional rehabilitation. The protocol explained on the extend of surgical treatment depending on the patient's severity, age as well as whether it can be done in stages or in combination to address the issues.

In multiple aims for rehabilitation in very young patient for example, increased ICP with hydrocephalus would necessitate less extensive surgical intervention such as ventriculoperitoneal (VP) shunting, while severe orbital proptosis might indicate temporary tarsorraphy, and respiratory difficulty would necessitate a continuous airway pressure device, a nasal stent, or a tracheostomy depending on the severity and the specific anatomic obstruction. More extensive surgical procedures are usually deferred up to certain age to reduce possibility of complications.

3.2.1 Posterior vault distraction/expansion

Posterior cranial vault expansion is usually indicated in increased in ICP cases without other functional issues when the patient's age is more suitable [26, 27]. The aim is to increase the cranial volume to accommodate for the brain growth whilst reducing the intra cranial pressure.

3.2.2 Fronto orbital advancement and Monobloc Le Fort III advancement

Increased ICP with orbital proptosis might require fronto-orbital advancement with or without cranioplasty, and increased ICP in the presence of orbital proptosis and hypoplastic maxilla might require a monobloc as practiced in the authors' center. Surgery can be performed conventionally or combined with distraction osteogenesis (DO) technique, which is indicated for superior structural expansion and achieving simultaneous new histogenesis compared with conventional surgical procedures [28]. The application of DO in treating craniofacial deformity was first reported in 1992 [29]. Since then, the benefits of this technique in treating syndromic craniosynostosis as reported in the literature are similar to those in the present study, which include marked improvements in functional parameters involving eye protection, preventing the increase of ICP, and treating airway deficiency [30–34].

3.2.3 Le Fort III osteotomy

Le Fort III advancement is aimed on improving the proptotic condition as well as opening the space for the upper airway. Syndromic craniosynostosis patients may presented with restricted upper airway thus causing obstructive sleep apnoea and shallow orbital floor. This allows the floor of the orbit to be advanced while opening the upper airway region on the nasal and maxillary region. This technique can be performed via conventional advancement or via DO depending on the amount of advancement and the experience of the team.

3.2.4 Le Fort I osteotomy

This is usually indicated in a later stage when the patient is more stable in growth to correct skeletal discrepancies such as retruded maxilla thus causing OSA. Therefore, the maxilla is advanced to gain space for airway. This procedure may be combined with other soft tissues surgery to gain optimum results in opening the airway such as tonsillectomy and adenoidectomy.

4. Complications

Craniofacial surgery is one of the established multidisciplinary specialty to produce safe surgery and good surgical outcome whilst minimizing the complications following surgical intervention for syndromic craniofacial patients. Although the results can be satisfying and there is general agreement on surgical indications, the potential remains for unwanted complications. The craniofacial surgery is unique because it involves exploration of the areas that allow very little margin of error. An inadequate knowledge of the anatomy, lack of training and surgical expertise can lead to not only disastrous results but even to the death of the patient. Any team that cares for craniofacial patients must take steps to avoid potential complications and be ready to deal with postoperative complications. Development of craniofacial surgery pioneered by Paul Tessier was a crucial step towards the paradigm shift in treating major craniofacial syndromic deformities [35].

4.1 Mortality and morbidity rate following craniofacial surgical intervention

The complications are the events that occurs during the management of craniofacial syndromes patients and may associated with any permanent deleterious effect on the patient. However, unfavourable outcomes generally are unexpected by the patients or surgeons [36].

The platinum rule to avoid any unwanted complications in any performed surgical procedures is to follow the dictum "Primum Non Nocere".

Many authors attempted to classify the complications of craniofacial surgery that arise during intraoperative and postoperative, but these complications might differ with different craniofacial syndromes. Intraoperative and post-operative complications pertaining to cranial vault surgery was described and classified into early, immediate post-operative and late postoperative complications [37–42]. Given the uniqueness presentation of patients with craniofacial syndromes, each patient presented with their own problems and complications following surgical intervention might be different from each other thus the need for comprehensive classification systems.

One of the easiest way to classify the complications following surgical intervention are by Sharma et al. 2013 [41] which was divided into four types:

Type 1: Minor events without any damaging effects on the patient. They include minor wound infections, poorly placed scars, minor cerebrospinal fluid leaks, and seromas/hematomas. Most of the time, this classification refers to less serious and minor complications following craniofacial surgery that consists of:

Epiphora

This is most of the time seen after hypertelorism correction but the reported incidence is quite low which is about 0.6% [42]. This is due to any procedure that involves dissection around the medial and inferomedial orbital floor may potentially damage the lacrimal drainage system.

Lateral canthal ligament dystopia

Extensive stripping of periorbita may lead to reattachment of periorbita at low level eventually resulting in enhanced antimongoloid slant. This is most frequently seen on syndromic rather than nonsyndromic craniofacial syndrome [22].

Hardware issues

Hardware can be considered as a foreign body thus occasionally can be infected, exposed or even palpable postoperatively. Infection and exposure of fixation material are rare in paediatric cranial vault surgery [42]. Metal fixation carry a possibility of intracranial fixation due to appositional cranial growth. Some reported translocation of hardware into calvarial bone in 14% and 6.6% with intracranial translocation and commonly occur in younger and syndromic patients [28]. Therefore, usage of resorbable hardware has now become more popular due to concerns about constriction of growth by metal fixation and the possibility of implant translocation [29–32].

Bone graft donor morbidity

Pneumothorax incidence of 3% after rib harvesting in their experience but emphasized that the rates vary from 5–30% in other series [33].

Type 2: Moderate-to-severe events that compromise the results and might need another surgical intervention for a successful outcome. They include exposure keratitis, diplopia, contour deformities, warping, non/malunion, and exposed hardware.

Strabismus and temporary ptosis are frequently seen after cranial vault procedures that involve periorbita stripping [37]. McCarthy et al. noted preoperative strabismus in hypertelorism cases, which often worsened after surgery then stabilized approximately 6 months after surgery [38].

Cerebrospinal fluid (CSF) leak following craniofacial surgery and sequalae of neurosurgical infection is common. Obvious risk for infection with CSF was noted but also associated with impairment of wound healing. Predisposing factor that might lead to easy tear of dura are due to scar from previous surgery or abnormal bony contour with dural adhesion [36–39]. Some tears may go unnoticed, and CSF may manifest postoperatively either as rhinorrhoea or leakage through the scalp wounds or within the drain itself.

Transient hyponatremia is one of the reported complications caused by secretion of inappropriate antidiuretic hormone (diabetes insipidus) has been reported [27, 40–44]. Researchers believe that it results from traction on the frontal lobes.

Unexpected airway issues are other complications following craniofacial surgery, in which emergency reintubation or even prolonged ventilation is needed due to severe upper airway oedema. Decision for steroid covers for upper airway oedema is most of the time anecdotal but some reported beneficial in preventing facial oedema postoperatively [45–50].

Type 3: Serious events with unfavourable result which can or cannot be successfully managed. They include nerve palsies and infection leading to bone loss and partial loss of vision.

Infection is the most common complication in the form of osteitis/osteomyelitis, meningitis, or an intracranial abscess, occurring in 6.2% of transcranial cases [25]. Overall reported infection rates ranging from 1–14% in large centre series [27, 32, 39–42, 47–51].

Permanent neurological deficit is another complication in craniofacial surgery that fall into type III classification. Majority of craniofacial surgery confined to extradural showed lower incidence of neurologic impairment. Several reports from major craniofacial centers has shown very low or no permanent neurologic deficits directly attributable to surgery [27, 30, 37, 50–52]. Blindness for example, is an unwanted complication in craniofacial surgery that post a real risk of blindness following surgery. Munro and Sabatier noted four cases of permanent blindness in 1092 procedures [54].

Type 4: Serious events that may even lead to death. They include postoperative infection, perioperative bleeding, respiratory compromise, or other serious anesthesia-related events.

Since 1970's to 1988, rate of mortality in craniofacial surgery were reported ranging from 1 to 2% all over the world [47–51]. However, with development of the technology, deeper understanding of the craniofacial surgery and its risks with emphasis on multidisciplinary approach, the numbers of mortality have dropped to 0.1–0.8% in some centers [24–29].

5. Research and development in corrective surgery

With the recent medical and technology advancement, patient management was more promising and in a well-controlled manner. The surgical management of craniosynostosis patient resurfaces again in the mid-20th century as a completely stand-alone surgical specialty. A more well defined surgical procedure, better anaesthetic protocols, together with the help of advanced technology, this group of patients now enjoy a safer surgical outcome [52–57].

5.1 Optimal age of surgery

Surgical procedures advocated in this group of patients are aim to make sure normal growth of the brain and skull, and near to normal development to their adulthood. Controversy still on-going with the best timing of surgical intervention in this group of patients between early versus late surgical intervention. Early surgical intervention is always aiming for better corneal protection and to create spaces for constricted brain. Late surgical intervention conversely aiming for more stable bony correction and less likely for subsequent surgical intervention [50]. However, our center practice on more indication and need-based approach, surgical intervention at the best possible timing for patients in term of growing stage, the indication need for the surgery and patient's general health condition [4].

5.2 Choices of osteotomy

Surgical procedures evolved from strip craniectomy, monobloc osteotomy, fronto orbital advancement and recently, posterior vault expansion. All these procedures are indicated to release the fused cranial suture, re-create more spaces for brain development and to make sure the bilateral eye globe is well protected as shown in **Figures 5** and **6**. The current treatment can be summarized in **Table 1**.

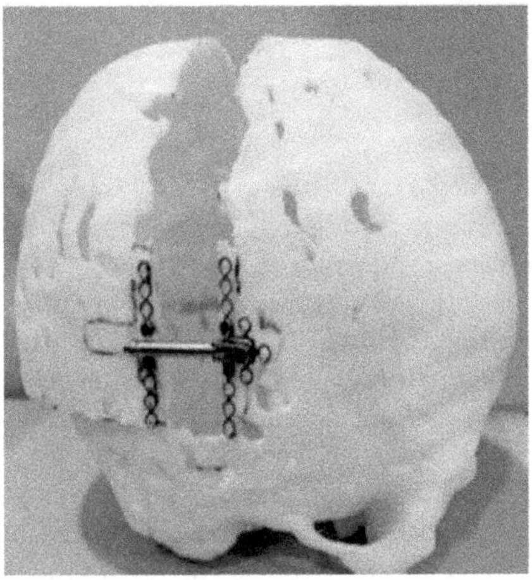

Figure 5.
Posterior vault distraction distraction osteogenesis indicated for only increased ICP with no other symptoms.

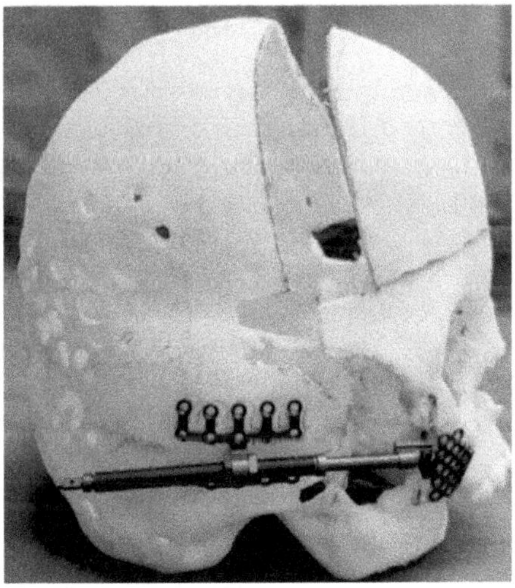

Figure 6.
Le Fort III advancement indicated for management of ICP, airway and orbital globe.

Issues to manage	Treatment proposed
Only increase in ICP	Posterior cranial vault distraction
Increase in ICP and shallow orbit	Fronto orbital advancement
Reduced airway and shallow orbit	Le Fort III advancement
Reduced airway, shallow orbit and increased ICP	Monobloc advancement

Table 1.
Treatment proposed for management of syndromic craniosynostosis issues.

Different surgeon will advocate different surgical technique at different timing, either with direct osteotomy and surgical plating or through distraction osteogenesis procedure [2, 4, 9, 49, 50, 58, 59]. There is no uniform surgical algorithm internationally, but more on surgeon or surgical center preferences. Obviously, these surgeries need collaboration of neurosurgeon, oral maxillofacial surgeon and otorhinolaryngologists.

5.3 Research

The ultimate goals for craniosynostosis treatment is mainly to restore function, improve facial aesthetic and ensure a healthy psychological development. More research is needed in this syndromic craniosynostosis in term of treatment algorithm, utilisation of latest and advancement of computer planning, computer navigation, 3-dimensional printing and usage of the cheaper, user friendly and effective surgical device in making the surgery more safer and more predictable outcome. The treatment focus not only on the fused suture of the skull, but also make an effort to address issue like intracranial pressure, strabismus, abnormally positioned orbit and dentofacial deformities [60–62]. Another area of future development will be in the molecular genetic testing in the field of genetic counselling.

6. Conclusions

Corrective surgery in syndromic craniosynostosis was formerly regarded as formidable however currently performed as a routine by major craniofacial center in the world due to advancement of technology and multidisciplinary approaches. Certain types of deformity, particularly those patients with Crouzon's or Apert's syndrome, require more than one functional intervention to achieve maximum correction.

In general, the surgical indication for paediatric CMF deformities can be classified into intermediate and definitive intervention. The intermediate intervention is performed at an early phase of patient's life and aimed to salvage vital tissue or organ function such as the brain, eye, airway or feeding which are essential for the child's development. The protocol of the management for syndromic craniosynostosis patients is summarized in **Figure** 7. These procedures include ventriculoperitoneal (VP) shunt, tarsorrhaphy, adenotonsillectomy and tracheostomy.

Therefore, these interventions in craniofacial syndromes is associated with multiple morbidities. It is important to understand the need and risks of these interventions prior making decision of treatment for each patient. Craniofacial teams should be cognizant to audit data on morbidity and mortality as well as surgical outcomes to monitor complication rates.

Surgical risk stratification involving the severity of patient's functional issues, age, co-morbidities, logistics, the timing and type of surgery and anticipated post-operative issues are in practiced to guide decision making consensus and serve as the index of precaution prior to any surgery [63]. This is in line with the recommendation of other centers which placed greater focus on protocols for airway management, blood salvage and replacement, age-appropriate deep venous thrombosis prophylaxis and timing of sub cranial midfacial advancements which might result in further reductions in craniofacial mortality rates.

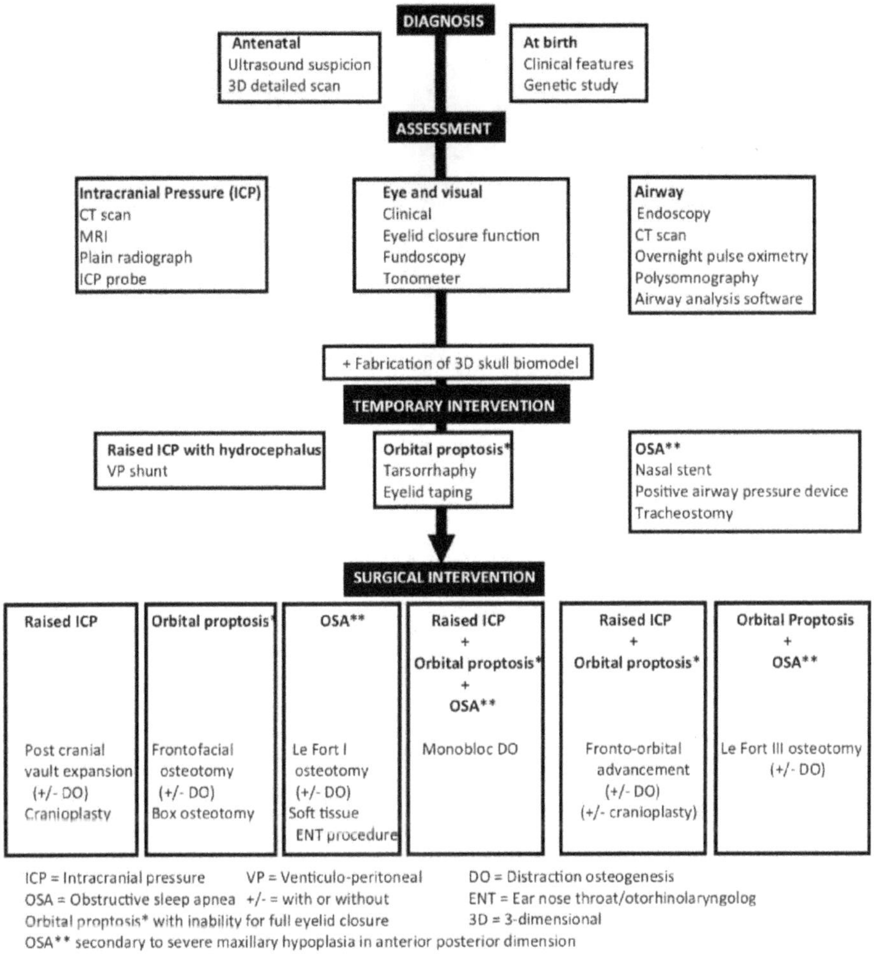

Figure 7.
Summary of indications for intervention in craniofacial syndromes.

Acknowledgements

We would like to thank everyone who were involved direct and indirectly in the making of this chapter, craniofacial team members, staff and patients in UMMC, HKL, and SASMEC@IIUM, Malaysia.

Conflict of interest

The authors declare no conflict of interest.

Author details

Khairul Bariah Chi Adam[1*], Firdaus Hariri[2], Wei Lee Chee[3], Kathiravan Purmal[4], Mohd Faizal Abdullah[5] and Nazer Berahim[6]

1 Oral Maxillofacial Surgery and Oral Diagnosis Department, Kulliyyah of Dentistry, International Islamic University Malaysia, Kuantan, Malaysia

2 Department of Oral and Maxillofacial Clinical Sciences, Faculty of Dentistry, University Malaya, Kuala Lumpur, Malaysia

3 Oral Maxillofacial Surgery Department, Hospital Kuala Lumpur, Malaysia

4 Katte Dental Clinic, Kuala Lumpur, Malaysia

5 School of Dental Sciences, Health Campus, Universiti Sains Malaysia, Kota Bharu, Malaysia

6 Oral Maxillofacial Surgery Department, Faculty of Dentistry, Universiti Teknologi MARA, Selangor, Malaysia

*Address all correspondence to: bariah@iium.edu.my

References

[1] Slater BJ, Lenton KA, Kwan MD, Gupta DM, Wan DC, Longaker MT. Cranial sutures: a brief review. Plastic and Reconstructive Surgery. 2008;**121**(4):170e-178e

[2] James CW, Laszlo N, Joshua CD. Syndromic craniosynostosis. Facial Plastic Surgery Clinics. 2016;**24**(4):531-543

[3] Gault DT, Renier D, Marchac D, Jones BM. Intracranial pressure and intracranial volume in children with craniosynostosis. Plastic and Reconstructive Surgery. 1992;**90**(3):377-381

[4] Hariri F, Azmi MN, Bahuri NF, Abdullah NA, Rahman ZA, Ganesan D. Crouzon syndrome: a case series of craniomaxillofacial distraction osteogenesis for functional rehabilitation. J Oral Maxillofac Surg. 2017;76(3):646.e1-646.e12.

[5] Kimonis V, Gold JA, Hoffman TL, Panchal J, Boyadjiev SA. Genetics of craniosynostosis. Seminars in Pediatric Neurology. 2007;**14**(3):150-161

[6] Wilkie AO, Bochukova EG, Hansen RM, et al. Clinical dividends from the molecular genetic diagnosis of craniosynostosis. American Journal of Medical Genetics. 1941;**143A**:200

[7] Laitinen L, Sulamaa M. Craniosynostosis; symptoms, treatment and results of treatment. II. Ann Paediatr Fenn. 1956;**2**(1):1-8

[8] Slater BJ, Lenton KA, Kwan MD, Gupta DM, Wan DC, Longaker MT. Cranial sutures: a brief review. Plast Reconstr Surg. 2008;121(4):170e – 8e.

[9] Gault DT, Renier D, Marchac D, Jones BM. Intracranial pressure and intracranial volume in children with craniosynostosis. Plastic and Reconstructive Surgery. 1992;**90**(3):377-381

[10] Derderian C, Seaward J. Syndromic craniosynostosis. Seminars in Plastic Surgery 2012;26(2):64-75.

[11] Bannink N, Joosten KFM, van Veelen M-LC, Bartels MC, Tasker RC, van Adrichem LNA, et al. Papilledema in patients with Apert, Crouzon, and Pfeiffer syndrome: prevalence, efficacy of treatment, and risk factors. The Journal of Craniofacial Surgery. 2008;**19**(1):121-127

[12] Johnson D, Wilkie AOM. Craniosynostosis. European Journal of Human Genetics. 2011;**19**(4):369-376

[13] Sharma VP, Fenwick AL, Brockop MS, McGowan SJ, Goos JAC, Hoogeboom AJM, et al. Mutations in TCF12, encoding a basic helix-loop-helix partner of TWIST1, are a frequent cause of coronal craniosynostosis. Nature Genetics. 2013;**45**(3):304-307

[14] Wilkie AOM, Byren JC, Hurst JA, Jayamohan J, Johnson D, Knight SJL, et al. Prevalence and complications of single-gene and chromosomal disorders in craniosynostosis. Pediatrics. 2010;**126**(2):e391-e400

[15] Renier D, Sainte-Rose C, Marchac D, Hirsch JF. Intracranial pressure in craniostenosis. Journal of Neurosurgery. 1982;**57**(3):370-377

[16] Thompson DN, Harkness W, Jones B, Gonsalez S, Andar U, Hayward R. Subdural intracranial pressure monitoring in craniosynostosis: its role in surgical management. Child's Nervous System. 1995;**11**(5):269-275

[17] Marucci DD, Dunaway DJ, Jones BM, Hayward RD. Raised intracranial pressure in Apert syndrome. Plastic and Reconstructive

Surgery. 2008;**122**(4):1162-1168 discussion 1169-1170

[18] Cornejo-Roldan LR, Roessler E, Muenke M. Analysis of the mutational spectrum of the FGFR2 gene in Pfeiffer syndrome. Human Genetics. 1999;**104**(5):425-431

[19] Muenke M, Schell U, Hehr A, Robin NH, Losken HW, Schinzel A, et al. A common mutation in the fibroblast growth factor receptor 1 gene in Pfeiffer syndrome. Nature Genetics. 1994;**8**(3):269-274

[20] Fearon JA, Rhodes J. Pfeiffer Syndrome: A Treatment Evaluation [Internet]. Vol. 123, Plast Reconstr Surg. 2009. p. 1560-1569. Available from: 10.1097/prs.0b013e3181a2057e.

[21] Adam KBC, Mahdah S, Azmi MN, Kadir K, Nabil S, Hariri F. Distraction osteogenesis in the craniomaxillofacial region. Part 1: History, principles, indications, types and protocol. Mal. Journal of Oral and Maxillofacial Surgery. 2014;**1**:1-7

[22] Al-Namnam NMN, Hariri F, Rahman ZAA. Distraction osteogenesis in the surgical management of syndromic craniosynostosis: a comprehensive review of published papers. The British Journal of Oral & Maxillofacial Surgery. 2018;**56**(5):353-366

[23] Hariri F, Kadir K, Nabil S, Abd Jabar MN, Samsudin AR, Rahman ZAA, et al. The use of 3-dimensional biomodel in planning paediatric craniofacial surgery. Mal J Oral Maxillofac Surg. 2014;**12**:8-13

[24] Cheung LK, Chua HDP, Hariri F, Lo J, Ow A, Zheng L. Chapter 30: Correction of Dentofacial Deformities. In M.A. Pogrel, K-E. Kahnberg & L. Andersson (Eds.), Essentials of Oral and Maxillofacial Surgery (pp. 315-330). Oxford, UK: Wiley Blackwell

[25] Greensmith AL, Meara JG, Holmes AD, Lo P. Complications related to cranial vault surgery. Oral and Maxillofacial Surgery Clinics of North America. 2004;**16**:465-473. DOI: 10.1016/j.coms.2004.07.001

[26] Hariri F, Ariff ZAR, Bahuri NF, Azmi MN. Distraction osteogenesis in Crouzon syndrome. J Oral Maxillofac Surg. 2018;76:646.e1-646.e12.

[27] McMillan K, Lloyd M, Evans M, et al. Experiences in performing posterior calvarial distraction. The Journal of Craniofacial Surgery. 2017;**28**:664

[28] Salokorpi N, Vuollo V, Sinikumpu JJ, et al: Increases in cranial volume with posterior cranial vault distraction in 31 consecutive cases. 2017;J Neurosurgery 81:803.

[29] Witherow H, Dunaway D, Evans R, et al. Functional outcomes in monobloc advancement by distraction using the rigid external distractor device. Plastic and Reconstructive Surgery. 2008;**121**:1311

[30] McCarthy JG, Schreiber J, Karp N, et al. Lengthening the human mandible by gradual distraction. Plastic and Reconstructive Surgery. 1992;**89**(1)

[31] Polley JW, Figueroa AA, Charbel FT, et al. Monobloc craniomaxillofacial distraction osteogenesis in a newborn with severe craniofacial synostosis: A preliminary report. The Journal of Craniofacial Surgery. 1995;**6**:421

[32] Shin JH, Duncan CC, Persing J. Monobloc distraction: Technical modification and considerations. The Journal of Craniofacial Surgery. 2003;**14**:763

[33] Yu W, Wang M, Yao K, et al. Individualized therapy for treating

obstructive sleep apnea in pediatric Crouzon syndrome patients. Sleep Breath J. 2016;**20**:1119

[34] Witherow H, Dunaway D, Evans R, et al. Functional outcomes in monobloc advancement by distraction using the rigid external distractor device. Plastic and Reconstructive Surgery. 2008;**121**:1311

[35] Tessier P. The definitive plastic surgical treatment of the severe facial deformities of craniofacial dysostosis, Crouzon's and Apert's disease. Plastic and Reconstructive Surgery. 1971;**48**:419-442

[36] Adam KB, Hariri F, Cheung LK, Nabil S, Aung LO, Rahman ZA. Technical Issues in Craniomaxillofacial Distraction Osteogenesis: A Case Series. Int Med J Malaysia. 2018;**17**:109-114

[37] Matthews D. Craniofacial surgery: indications, assessment and complications. British Journal of Plastic Surgery. 1979;**32**(2):96-105. DOI: 10.1016/0007-1226(79)90006-7

[38] McCarthy JG, Thorne CHM, Wood-Smith D. Principles of craniofacial surgery: orbital hypertelorism. In: McCarthy JG, editor. Plastic surgery Cleft lip and palate and craniofacial anomalies. Vol. 4. WB Saunders; 1990. p. 2974-3012.

[39] Marchac D, Renier D. Complications. In: Marchac D, Reiner D, editors. Craniofacial surgery for craniosynostosis. Boston. Little: Brown and Company; 1982. p. 176

[40] Kirkpatrick WN, Koshy CE, Waterhouse N, Fauvel NJ, Carr RJ, Peterson DC. Paediatric transcranial surgery: a review of 114 consecutive procedures. British Journal of Plastic Surgery. 2002;**55**:561-564

[41] Sharma RK. Unfavourable results in craniofacial surgery. Indian J Plast Surg. 2013;**46**:204-214

[42] Whitaker LA, Munro IR, Salyer KE, Jackson IT, Ortiz-Monasterio F, Marchac D. Combined report of problems and complications in 793 craniofacial operations. Plastic and Reconstructive Surgery. 1979;**64**:198

[43] Levine JP, Stelnicki E, Weiner H, Bradley JP, McCarthy JG. Hyponatraemia in the postoperative craniofacial pediatric patient population: a connection to cerebral salt wasting syndrome and management of the disorder. Plastic and Reconstructive Surgery. 2001;**108**:1501-1508

[44] Steig PE, Mulliken JB. Neurosurgical complications in craniofacial surgery. Neurosurgery Clinics of North America. 1991;**2**:703-708

[45] Habal MB. Prevention of postoperative facial oedema with steroids after facial surgery. Aesthetic Plastic Surgery. 1985;**9**:69-71

[46] Neil-Dwyer JG, Evans RD, Jones BM, Hayward RD. Tumescent steroid infiltration to reduce postoperative swelling after craniofacial surgery. British Journal of Plastic Surgery. 2001;**54**:565-569

[47] Israele V, Siegel JD. Infectious complications of craniofacial surgery in children. Reviews of Infectious Diseases. 1989;**11**:9-15

[48] David DJ, Poswillo DE, Simpson DA. The craniosynostoses:causes, natural history and management.Berlin7. Springer-Verlag; 1982

[49] Taylor JA, Bartlett SP. What's new in syndromic craniosynostosis surgery? Plastic and Reconstructive Surgery. 2017;**140**:82e-93e

[50] Proctor MR, Meara JG. A review of the management of single -suture craniosynostosis, past, present, and future. Journal of Neurosurgery. Pediatrics. 2019;**24**:622-631

[51] Cerisola J, Rohwedder R. Bacterial contamination of the operating field in craniofacial surgery: a new schedule of antibiotic prophylaxis. In: Transactions of the Eighth International Congress of Plastic and Reconstructive Surgery. Montreal. 1983. p. 283-285.

[52] Sebatier R, Munro IR', Lauritzen C. A review of two thousand craniomaxillofacial operations. In: Transactions of the Eighth International Congress of Plastic and Reconstructive Surgery. Montreal. 1983. p. 329-30

[53] Whitaker LA, Munro IR, Jackson IT, Salyer KE. Problems in cranio-facial surgery. Journal of Maxillofacial Surgery. 1976;**4**:131

[54] Converse JM, Wood-Smith D, McCarthy JG. Report on a series of 50 craniofacial operations. Plastic and Reconstructive Surgery. 1975;**55**:283

[55] Poole MD. Complications in craniofacial surgery. British Journal of Plastic Surgery. 1988;**41**:608

[56] Kececi Y, Ozek C, Gurler T, et al. Complications in craniofacial surgery: the Turkish experience. The Journal of Craniofacial Surgery. 2000;**11**(2):168-171. DOI: 10.1097/00001665-200011020-00012

[57] Jones BM, Jani P, Bingham RM, Mackersie AM, Hayward R. Complications in paediatric craniofacial surgery: an initial four year experience. British Journal of Plastic Surgery. 1992;**45**:225-231

[58] David DJ, Cooter RD. Craniofacial infection in 10 years of transcranial surgery. Plastic and Reconstructive Surgery. 1987;**80**:213-223

[59] Munro IR, Sabatier RE. An analysis of 12 years of craniomaxillofacial surgery in Toronto. Plastic and Reconstructive Surgery. 1985;**76**:29

[60] Yilmaz E, Mihci E, Nur B, Alper ÖM, Taçoy Ş. Recent Advances in Craniosynostosis. Pediatric Neurology. 2019;**99**:7-15

[61] Guimarães-Ferreira J, Miguéns J, Lauritzen C. Advances in Craniosynostosis Research and Management. Advances and Technical Standards in Neurosurgery. 2004; 23-83.

[62] Mahdah S, Bariah K, Azmi MN, Saleh I, Nabil S, Hariri F. Distraction osteogenesis in the craniomaxillofacial region. Part II: Peri-operative issues, surgical procedure, complications and reliability. Mal. Journal of Oral and Maxillofacial Surgery. 2015;**13**(1):1-10

[63] Hariri F, Abdullah MF, Adam KB, Bahuri NF et. al. Analysis of complications following multidisciplinary functional intervention in paediatric crnaiomaxillofacial deformities. 2019. Int J Oral Maxillofac. DOI: 10.1016/j. ijom.2020.08.02

Chapter 8

Telescoping with Multiple Revolution Cranial Osteotomies in Patients with Simple Craniosynostosis

Diego José Caycedo, Marcela Cabal Castro and Luís Fernando Santacruz

Abstract

Simple craniosynostosis is a cranial deformity that occurs secondary to a premature closure of one or more sutures, with a consequent alteration in cranial growth and cerebral expansion. The cranial alteration presents as flattening parallel to the compromised suture, with compensatory bulging in a perpendicular vector. The surgical treatment consists in cranial decompressions with suturectomies and simultaneous cranioplasties. Dynamic multiple revolution osteotomies allow the design of bone flaps that can help with decompression and correct secondary deformities caused by the synostosis. This multicenter descriptive case series study assessed 52 patients (12 plagiocephaly, 29 scaphocephaly, 7 brachycephaly and 4 trigonocephaly) operated in Cali, Colombia. In each case, suturectomy and telescoping with multiple revolution cranial osteotomies were designed to correct each particular deformity. No clinical complications were observed in the postoperative period (1, 90, and 180 days), and excellent outcomes with no re ossification of sutures and maintenance of the cranioplasty, based on clinical observation and findings in the 3D reconstruction scans.

Keywords: telescoping, osteotomies, cranioplasty, suturectomy, craniosynostosis

1. Introduction

Simple craniosynostosis is a cranial deformity that occurs secondary to a premature closure of one or more sutures, with a consequent alteration in cranial growth and cerebral expansion. It develops during the first years of life and affects 1 in every 2000 to 2500 births worldwide [1]. The cranial alteration presents as flattening parallel to the compromised suture, with compensatory bulging in a perpendicular vector [2, 3].

The surgical treatment consists in cranial decompressions with suturectomies and simultaneous cranioplasties. Dynamic multiple revolution osteotomies allow the design of bone flaps that can help with decompression and correct secondary deformities caused by the synostosis. This multicenter descriptive case series study assessed 52 patients (12 plagiocephaly, 29 scaphocephaly, 7 brachycephaly and 4 trigonocephaly) operated in Cali, Colombia. In each case, suturectomy and telescoping with multiple revolution cranial osteotomies were designed to correct each particular deformity. No clinical complications were observed in the postoperative period (1, 90, and 180 days), and excellent outcomes with no re ossification of sutures and maintenance of the cranioplasty, based on clinical observation and findings in the 3D reconstruction scans.

Craniosynostosis surgical techniques have evolved over time. Initially extensive craniotomies with or without the use of alloplastic substances between bone gaps were described to release de compromised suture and allow cerebral decompression. Uncertain and inconsistent results were observed, that usually required reoperations and ended in poor esthetic results [4–7]. Developing techniques included the addition of bone remodeling for the compensatory defects using cranial bone grafts (static remodeling) and the use of different osteosynthesis materials. Given the evidence around the rapid ossification during the first year of life, nowadays gradual osteogenic distraction is one of the preferred procedures associated to skull osteotomies and cranial bone flap remodeling [8]. Osteotomies that remove bone segments and relocate them as bone grafts for cranial remodeling, increase the possibility of complications due to dead space formation between dura mater and bone grafts [9].

Over time, distraction osteogenesis has become very important in the surgical treatment of craniosynostosis. In 1998, Lauritzen et al. [10] proposed the dynamic cranial remodeling technique with expansive springs, placed between the osteotomies (without dural dissection) thereby promoting expansive forces that prevented deformity recurrence. Salyer & Bardach [11] proposed, for the correction of scaphocephaly, posterior bi-parietal osteotomies molding bone grafts after separating them from the skull. Similar proposals were made by Tullous et al. [12] and Solís-Salgado & Anaya-Jara [13]. Cardim [14] presented excellent results with the use of springs and dynamic osteotomies (Nautilus), however, the maintenance of postoperative expansion was sometimes affected by the scalp flap or by positional effects.

The primary aim and motivation of our craniofacial surgery team in Cali, Colombia, is to find a stable maintenance option of the postoperative expanded shape. The proposal is to maintain the bone expansion achieved by telescoping (dynamic spiral) osteotomies with 2-center spirals, by placing absorbable plates at 180 degrees from each other, arranging them with a level-based organization according to each circumvolution (**Figure 1**).

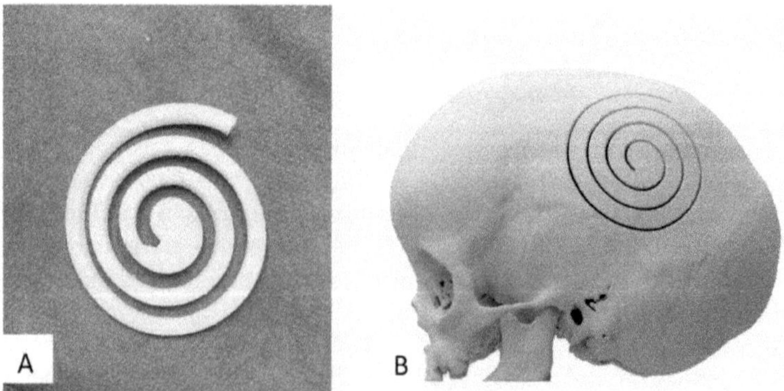

Figure 1.
(A) 2 centered spiral shape; (B) Representation of the spiral osteotomies.

2. Classification of Craniosynostosis

Two methods of classifications of craniosynostosis are used: anatomical and etiological. Anatomical classifications identify the fused cranial suture. There are four major sutures, and they can be altered as single metopic or sagittal sutures or as paired coronal and lambdoid sutures.

Single suture synostosis most commonly involve the sagittal suture (45%), followed by coronal (22%), metopic (22%), and lambdoid (5%). Alternatively, an etiological classification emphasizes the primary cause of craniosynostosis. The two most common causes of craniosynostosis are restriction of fetal head movement during pregnancy and single gene disorders that predispose to suture fusion. Bilateral coronal and multiple suture synostosis occur with disproportionate frequency in syndromic cases.

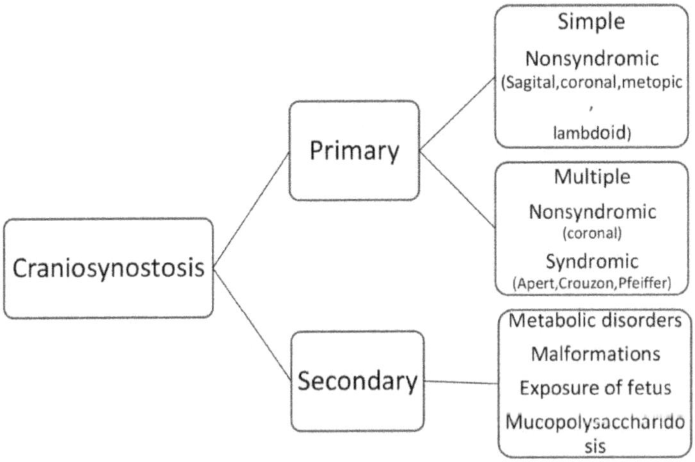

3. Presurgical preparation

The indications for surgery and inclusion criteria were patients diagnosed with simple craniosynostosis without previous surgical treatment and who had evident cranial deformity verified with X-ray and tomography. Children between 3 months and 4 years old. Excluded patients were those with syndromic craniosynostosis, children with previous surgical treatments, and patients with indication of minimally invasive cranial correction.

A multidisciplinary medical group consisting of a plastic surgeon, pediatric neurosurgeon and anesthesiologist asses all patients. To support the best surgical plan, 3D imaging Ct scans are performed. Its required to guarantee for all patients a strict monitoring of the anesthesia including colocation of central catheter, arterial route, bladder catheter ant temperature monitoring. It's also required to have guaranteed intraoperative blood transfusion. After the intervention all patients are transferred to intensive care unit. The first follow up of the patients are done every 3 months and then 3 more follow ups every 6 months until the second year after the interventions.

Patients that had cranioplasty surgery with a telescopic osteotomy, were divided in subgroups according to their alterations for surgical purposes. These subgroups are: Diagnosis of scaphocephaly, brachyophaly, plagiocephaly, and trigonecephaly. Patients with the scaphocephaly diagnosis are intervined with the "PI" technique and in the bi-temporoparietal regions, multiple- revolutions oseotomies were used to achieve the expansion and telescoping of osteotomies. Absorbable plates are staggered in three levels with a 180 degree in each circumvolution within the dynamic osteotomy. Patients with plagiocephaly, brachycephaly and trigonocephaly were treated with corticotomy surgeries for the liberation of the synostosed sutures and with dynamic osteotomies depending on the altered areas, fixing plates in the same alternating form as described previously for scaphocephaly

4. Surgical technique

Patients underwent general anesthesia, with endotracheal intubation and bilateral tarsorrhaphy, and placed in supine decubitus on the surgical table. A zigzag shape bitemporal coronal incision was made and a subsequent subperiosteally dissection was performed until the compromised suture was completely exposed.

In patients with scaphocephaly, the synostosis was managed with a "PI" technique osteotomy (**Figure 2**), removing the bone segments on each side of the sagittal suture. Then sub cranial dissection in the temporal regions was performed, as well as design of spiral osteotomies (**Figure 3**). With and without mechanical traction of the bone flaps of the spiral osteotomies, decompression was observed. (**Figure 4**). To maintain the expansion and telescoping of the osteotomies, at each level of the spiral absorbable plates were placed at each level of the spiral at 180 degrees from each other (**Figure 5**). This allows the lasting cranial decompression observed in the 3-d Computerized Tomography scan (**Figure 6**).

In plagiocephaly, brachycephaly and trigonocephaly cases (**Figure 7**), after the release of the compromised suture, spiral osteotomy was performed in the flattened areas of the skull. After checking the adequate release of the suture, the absorbable plate was placed to maintain telescoping (expansion) (**Figure 8**). The patients in the immediate postoperative period were transferred to the intensive care unit (ICU) for 2 days and then to a hospitalization room for 4 to 5 days.

5. Clinical evaluation

The patients that met the inclusion criteria were determined by a clinical evaluation. Out of the 52 diagnosed patients with simple craniosynostosis, 12 were plagiocenphaly, 29 scaphacephaly, 7 brachycephaly and 4 trigonocephaly. The average age of patients was 16.3 months. No mayor complications were observed in the intra operative and post - operative stage. No seromas, cerebrospinal fluid fistula or signs of infections. Only in two patients, the formation of granuloma was observed at the incisions and was resolved with the suture removal. In the neurological recurrent assessment, none of the patients showed any alteration and there was no suspicion of Intracranial Hypertension recurrence according to clinical charts. Furthermore, none of the patients had an increased hospitalization time in the intensive care unit or in the ward. .3D CT scans were requested to all patients for evaluation of the surgical procedure at different times (**Figure 6**). In all patients, correction of the cranial deformity in the immediate postoperative period was observed (**Figures 7–9**). Likewise, the results were maintained over time and they were assessed at the controls after 3 and 6 months of surgery (**Figure 9**).

The craniofacial surgery team and their families judged the results in follow ups that went from 6 to 25 months after surgery. Sixteen of the patients had an excellent aesthetical correction of their deformities. In 4 cases the family was pleased with the outcomes, but the craniofacial surgery team identifies mild residual deformity.

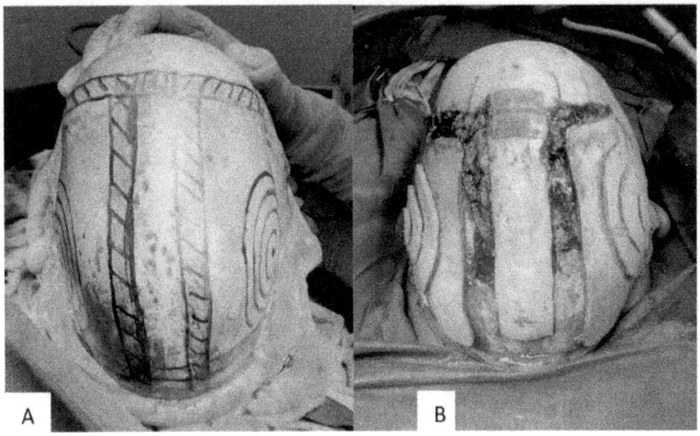

Figure 2.
Intraoperative images of a scaphocephaly correction; (A) Intrasurgical suturectomies design; (B) "PI" shape modification osteotomy.

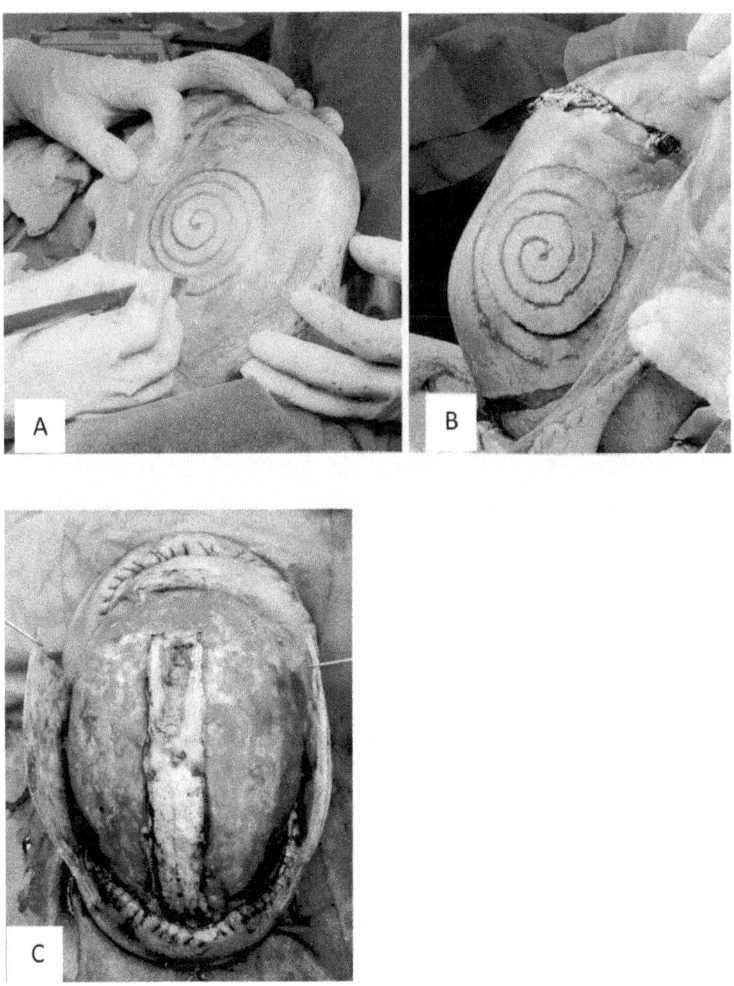

Figure 3.
Intraoperative images of a scaphocephaly correction. (A) Design of technique, (B) Spiral osteotomies, and (C) Sub-cranial dissection.

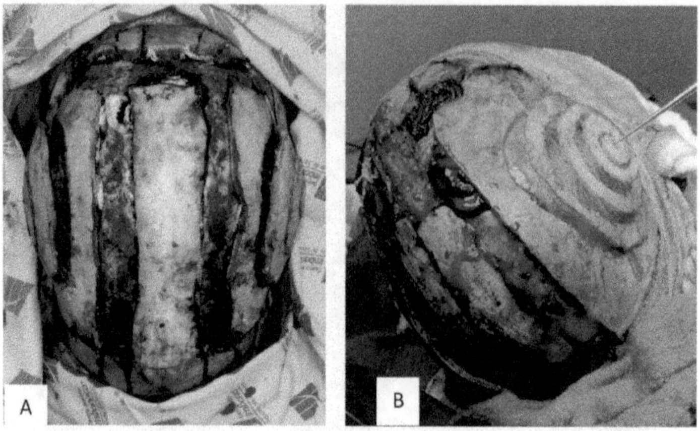

Figure 4.
Superior image view of the spiral osteotomy in a scaphocephaly correction. (A) Osteotomy without applied traction; (B) osteotomy with traction.

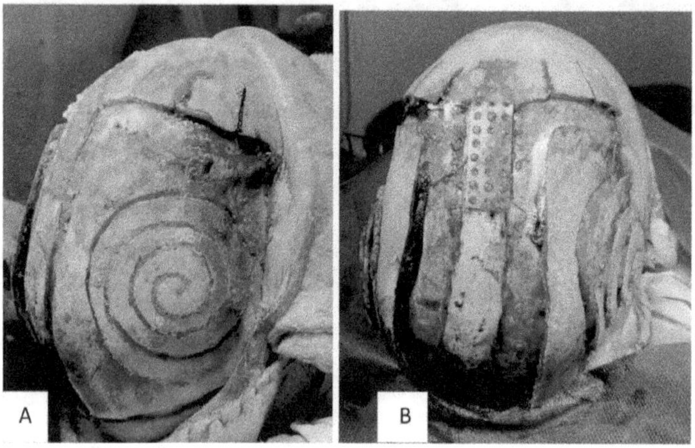

Figure 5.
Scaphocephaly correction. (A) View of the lateral intraoperative spinal osteotomy with absorbable plates places al 180. (B) Intraoperative superior view.

6. Discussion

In simple craniosynostosis, cranial alterations are the result of skull compensation to the premature closure of a suture. This deformity allows adequate brain growth to avoid neurological sequelae resulting from compression of structures. According to Virchow descriptions [2, 3], different cranial shapes can be found depending on the suture alteration.

The aim of the different surgical procedures described for the synostosis correction is to provide predictable and stable outcomes and the prevention of neurological changes, secondary to cerebral compression. All surgical plans including craniectomies, suturectomies, subsequent reconstruction procedures [4, 5] and the use of cranial expansion devices or any ostheosynthesis material [6, 7] need to consider the least traumatic choice for the patient and consider always that unexpected morbidities can present.

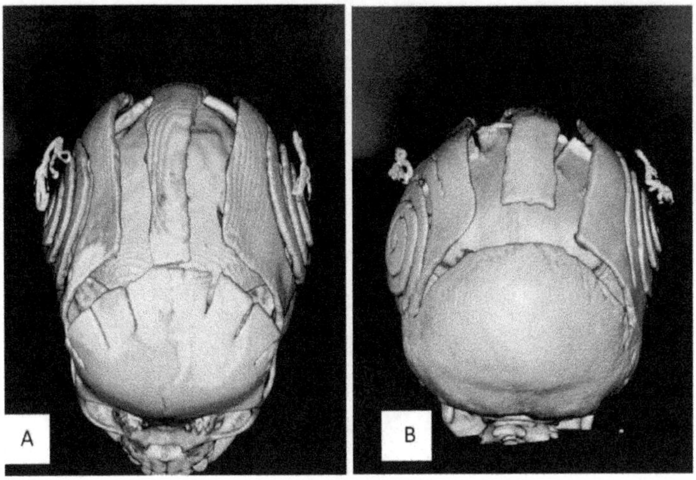

Figure 6.
3-D computerized tomography (CT) scan, it was taken on the 2nd postoperative day: (A) Superior view. (B) Posterior view.

Protection of the dura and the brain is achieved with the spiral craniotomies or dynamic revolution procedure, therefore lowering the morbidity rates. This advantage can also be observed when combining skull and facial procedures, as it's indicated in the treatment of syndromic craniosynostosis [9]. By designing bone flaps in spiral osteotomies [10, 12], the correction of the deformity has successful and stable outcomes. Also allowing adequate expansion of the brain in a more uniform, progressive way and obtaining a more anatomical shape [13, 14].

In general, it is considered that treatment should be carried out at an early age, from the third month to the first year of life [15, 16]. These osteotomies do not separate the dura from the calotte, thereby avoiding dead spaces that can allow seromas that usually complicate the craniosynostosis surgical intervention [17].

This craniotomy technique focused on keeping a stable expansion of the structures, which helps enhance the healing process. Therefore, the hypothesis was that the maintenance of expansion after the replacement and closure of the scalp flap, and despite the compression of the child's head support (e.g. at sleep), should improve esthetic and functional surgical outcomes. This study aims to contribute to the answer of two questions: how to achieve stable bone distraction and expansion. And how to perform in a simple and practical way the telescoping surgery technique by involving absorbable plates at 180 degrees from each other in the circular osteotomy (**Figure 5**).

This proposed technique has several advantages. This technique allows patients under 4-years to be treated by this surgical technique for simple craniosynostosis. It allows the brain and the skull to grow in a natural and symmetric way while having a protective frame achieved by the absorbable plates. Managing less neurological risks while obtaining a more dynamic skull growth. However, this technique is also invasive as previously described techniques. Performing the osteotomies with the expected circumvolutions requires expertise, practice of the technique is suggested before incorporating it in order to master and avoid complications. Although this technique is time consuming, no additional disadvantages or complications have been found in comparison with regular craniosynostosis procedures.

There are various techniques for cranial remodeling described in the literature for each type of craniosynostosis. Each technique has its advantages and

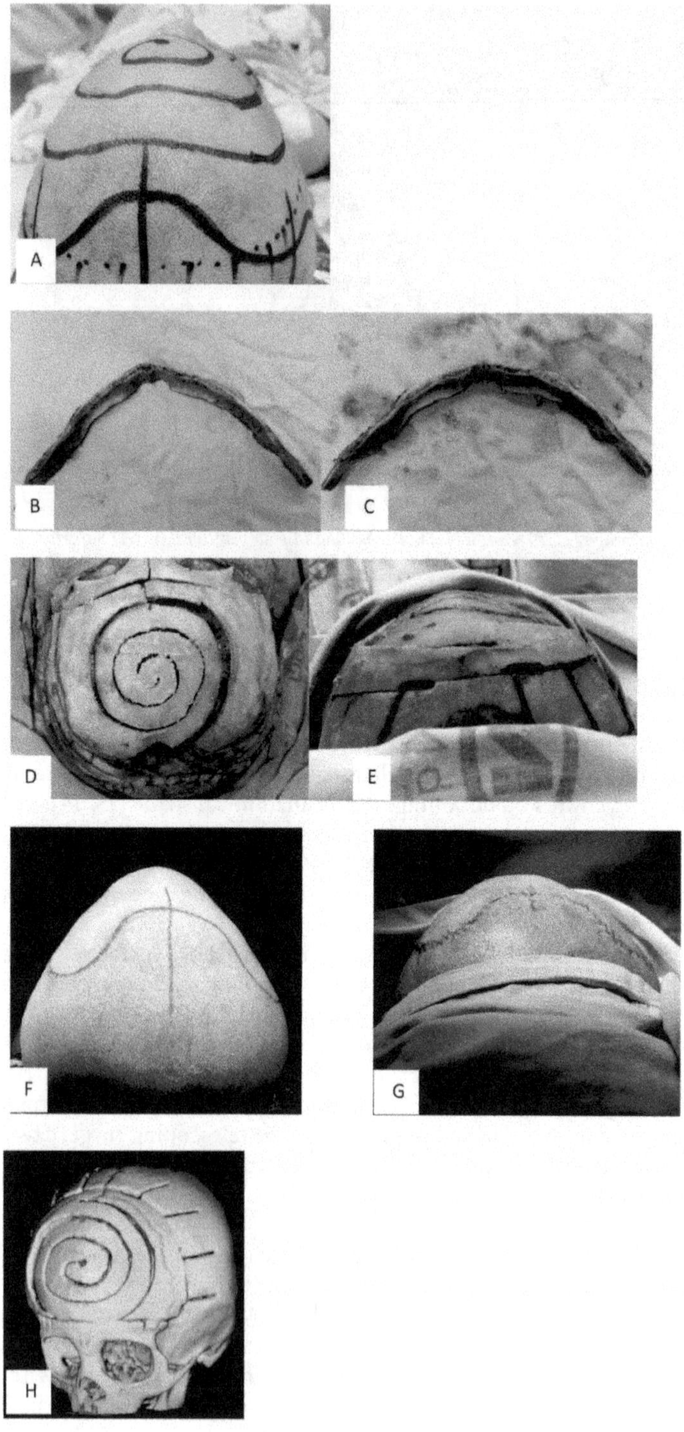

Figure 7.
Trigonocephaly correction. (A): Pre-surgical plan, (B) Fronto-orbital bar, (C) Remodeled frontoorbital bar, (D, E): Superior and frontal intraoperative views of the osteotomy showing the spiral design. (F) Preoperative, (G) Postoperative, (H) Post- surgical 3-D computerized tomography (CT).

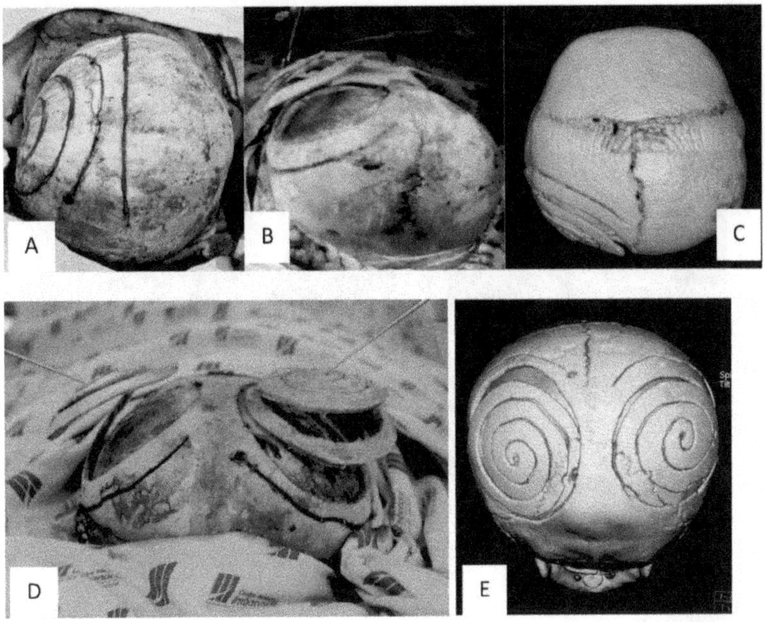

Figure 8.
Posterior plagiocephaly cases. (A) Pre-surgical plan for posterior plagiocephaly (B) Intraoperative image osteotomies showing the spiral design (C) Post- surgical 3-D computerized tomography (CT) (D) Intraoperative osteotomies for posterior plagiocephaly, showing treatment of the lambdoidea suture with the spiral bilateral shape (E) Post- surgical 3-D computerized tomography (CT).

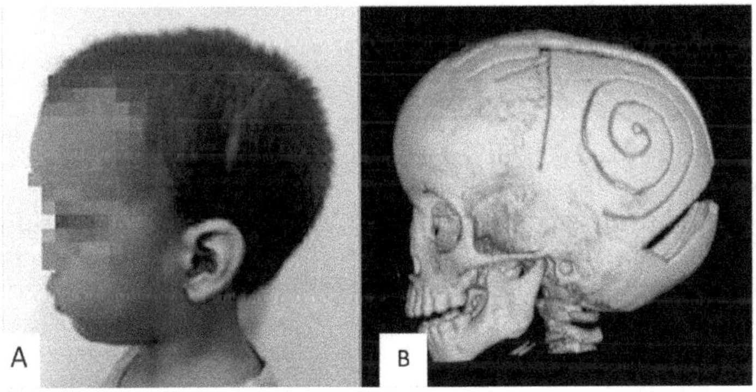

Figure 9.
(A) Scaphocephaly case, 3rd month post- surgical control, (B) 3-D computerized tomography (CT).

disadvantages. The idea of the proposed dynamic spiral craniotomies is to add other alternative to the different existing tools and to analyze its advantages.

For anterior plagiocephaly what is usually described is a unilateral fronto-orbital bar advancement that allows for the correction of asymmetries and retrusion of the orbits. For the frontal flattening and bossing of each side, what has been described is a craniectomy with cranioplasty and repositioning of each segment as bone grafts. With the spiral osteotomies what can be achieved is the correction of both the flattening and bossing, without the need of craniectomies, preserving the bone as flaps, thus conserving its vascularization and needing less dissection. These diminish the risk of comorbidities associated to greater dura detachments. For

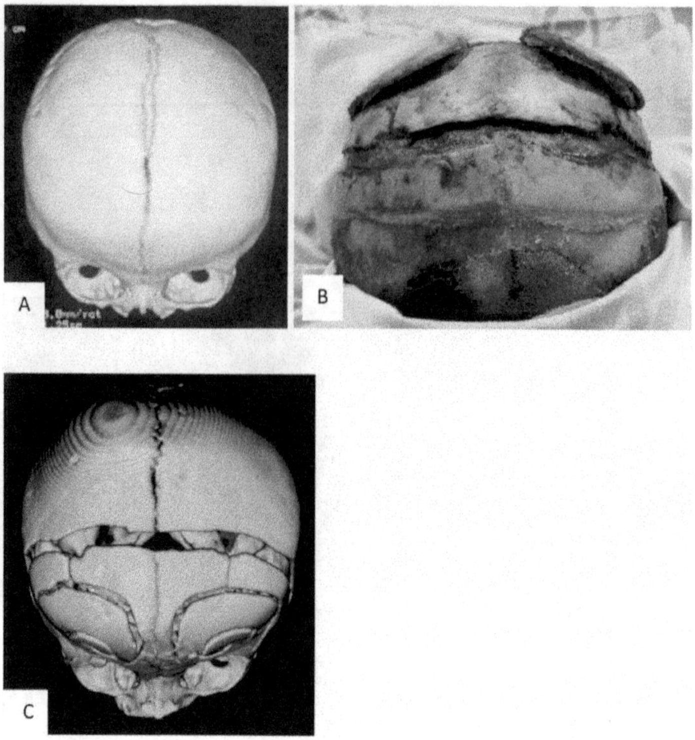

Figure 10.
Anterior brachycephaly. (A) Pre- surgical 3-D computerized tomography (CT) (B) Intraoperative view of osteotomies for coronal suturectomy and bilateral spiral osteotomies (C) Post-surgical 3-D computerized tomography (CT) superior view.

brachycephaly the technique is very similar, but the goal is to correct the flattening in both sides of the frontal bone (**Figure 10**). In posterior plagiocephaly what the literature has described for correction is the Mercedes technique, but it is associated to high complication rates for being highly traumatic and for long surgical times. With the lambdoid decompression associated to the dynamic osteotomies the functional and occipital asymmetries can be corrected with less complication rates (**Figure 8**). In trigonocephaly spiral osteotomies are also an alternative to allow for the remodeling of the frontal bone without the need of craniectomies and wide dissections (**Figure 7**).

As shown, spiral osteotomies firstly described in literature by Tullous in 2001 can be considered a useful tool for the treatment of all of the different synostosis deformities, as an alternative that conserves the vascularization of cranial bones, lowering the needs of greater dissections and craniectomies, and lowering surgical times and comorbidities. It is an option that has shown results that last over time (**Figure 11**).

7. Conclusions

The surgical correction via simple craniosynostosis with spiral osteotomies allows the achievement of cranial expansion with low morbidity rates. The results were that the skull areas where the osteotomies were performed, showed that tat they have their own vascularization, acting as bone flaps that enhanced the healing

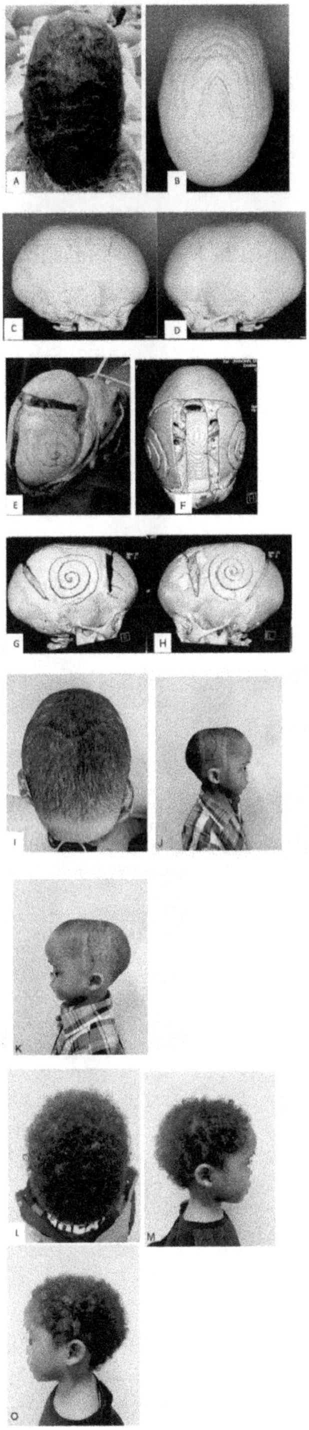

Figure 11.
(A) Scaphocephaly preoperative picture and (B-D) the 3D computerized tomography (CT), (E) Intraoperative view showing craniectomies and the marking of the spiral osteotomies in the parietal bones, (F-H) Pos surgical 3-D computerized tomography (CT), (I-K) 3 weeks pos surgical control, L,M,N: 2 and a half years post-surgical control.

process and diminished risks of seroma formation. In addition, a normal and natural development of the skull shape is achieved by the protection given by the absorbable plates in each spiral convolution of the osteotomies performed. Allowing it to maintain the surgical success over time (3 to 6 months).

Conflict of interest

The authors declare no conflict of interests regarding their current affiliations, besides the institutions where the present study was carried out.

Author details

Diego José Caycedo[1,2]*, Marcela Cabal Castro[1,2] and Luís Fernando Santacruz[2]

1 Division of Plastic and Reconstructive Surgery, Valle University "Universidad del Valle" Medical School, Colombia

2 Imbanaco Medical Center "Centro Médico Imbanaco". "Fundación Club Noel" Children´s Clinic, Cali, Colombia

*Address all correspondence to: diego.caycedo@imbanaco.com.co, diegojosecaycedo@gmail.com and www.diegocaycedo.com

References

[1] Slater, B. J., Lenton, K. A., Kwan, M. D., Gupta, D. M., Wan, D. C., & Longaker, M. T. (2008). Cranial sutures: a brief review. Plastic and reconstructive surgery, 121(4), 170e-178e.

[2] Persing JA, Jane JA, Shaffrey M. Virchow and the pathogenesis of craniosynostosis: a translation of his original work. *Plast Reconstr Surg.* 1989;83(4):738-42.

[3] Mark ES, Persing JA, Christopher I, Shaffrey JAJ. Craniosynostosis. In: Rengachary SS, Wilkins RH, eds. *Principles of neurosurgery. 2nd ed. London:* Wolfe; 2004. p.8.2-8.15.

[4] Lannelongue M. De la Craniectomie dans la microcephalie. *C R Acad Sci* Paris.1890; 110:1382-1385.

[5] Lane L. Pioneer craniectomy for relief of mental imbecility due to premature sutural losure and microcephalus. *JAMA*.1892; 18: 49-50

[6] Guimarães-Ferreira J, Miguens J, Lauritzen C. Advances in craniosynostosis research and management. *Adv Tech Stand Neurosurg.* 2004;29:23-83.

[7] Greensmith AL, Holmes AD, Lo P, Maxiner W, Heggie AA, Meara JG. Complete correction of severe scaphocephaly: the Melbourne method of total vault remodeling. *Plast Reconstr Surg.* 2008;121(4):1300-10.

[8] Cardim VLN, Dornelles RFV. Craniossinostoses. In: Carreirão S, Carneiro Jr. LVF, eds. *Cirurgia plástica para a formação do especialista.* São Paulo: Atheneu; 2011. p.297-308.

[9] Ortiz-Monasterio F, del Campo AF, Carrillo A. Advancement of the orbits and the midface in one piece, combined with frontal repositioning, for the correction of Crouzon's deformities. *Plast Reconstr Surg.* 1978;61(4):507-16.

[10] Lauritzen C, Sugawara Y, Kocabalkan O, Olsson R. Spring mediated dynamic craniofacial reshaping. Case report. *Scand J Plast Reconstr Surg Hand Surg.* 1998;32(3):331-8.

[11] Salyer KE, Bardach J. *Salyer & Bardach's atlas of craniofacial & cleft surgery.* Philadelphia: Lippincott-Raven; 1999.

[12] Tullous MW, Henry MN, Wang PTH, Vollmer DG, Auber AE, Mancuso PA. Multiple-revolution spiral osteotomy for cranial reconstruction. Technical note. *J Neurosurg.* 2001;94(4):671-6.

[13] Solís-Salgado O, Anaya-Jara M. Remodelación craneal para craneosinostosis sagital mediante osteotomía en forma de espiral usando sistema de fijación con miniplacas y tornillos absorbibles. *Arch Neurocien.* 2009;14(4):221 30.

[14] Cardim VLN, Silva AS, Salomons RL, Dornelles RFV, Lima e Silva A, Blom JOS, Zanon Colange N. Nautilus: craniotomia dinâmica - nova técnica cirúrgica e resultados preliminares, *Rev Bras Cir Plas;* 2013; 28(1): 29-35.

[15] Panchal J, Uttchin V. Management of craniosynostosis. *Plast Reconstr Surg.* 2003;111(6):2032-48.

[16] Cohen MMJ. Craniosynostosis: diagnosis, evaluation and management. *New York: Raven Press;* 1986.

[17] Cardim VLN, Silva AS, Salomons RL, Dornelles RFV, Lima e Silva A, Blom JOS. Remodelagem de crânios maduros utilizando molas expansoras. *Rev Bras Cir Craniomaxilofac.* 2012;15(2):57-63.

www.ingramcontent.com/pod-product-compliance
Lightning Source LLC
LaVergne TN
LVHW061911211125
826084LV00006B/684